Becoming a Successful Scholar

Guido Filler • Ravneet Nagra

Becoming a Successful Scholar

A Practical Guide to Academic Achievement in the Medical Professions

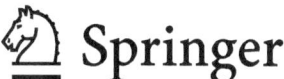 Springer

Guido Filler
Western University
London, ON
Canada

Ravneet Nagra
Western University
London, ON
Canada

ISBN 978-3-030-24447-7   ISBN 978-3-030-24448-4   (eBook)
https://doi.org/10.1007/978-3-030-24448-4

This Springer imprint is published by the registered company Springer
Nature Switzerland AG
The registered company address is: Gewerbestrasse 11, 6330 Cham, Switzerland

Contents

Chapter 1
Introduction

We live in a world of high change and uncertainty. Things change at an incredible pace. As the "baby boomers" are on their way out of the job market, their children are entering it, and the competitiveness that their parents experienced is now facing them. Are you feeling threatened by this competitiveness? Then this book is for you!

What is a baby boomer? It is a term for a demographic cohort, representing the birth years of approximately the mid-1940s to mid-1960s. The phrase reflects the significant increase in the birth rate after World War II. Traditionally, they have been associated with a rejection or redefinition of traditional values. However, I don't believe that. Typically, the values of all generations eventually become the same. The high birth rates resulted in substantial competition during school, university, and of course in the job market. It was a struggle to get the desired job. As a consequence, baby boomers embraced the competition. Achieving success in the job became of utmost importance to them. They are all about achievement and legacy. The end of the baby boomer years is marked by the introduction of the contraceptive pill in the mid-1960s, which led to a dramatic decline in the birth rate.

The following generation is Generation X or the "Gen-Xers." They reflect the birth years of approximately 1965–1985. The dramatic fall in the birth rate leads to rather differing job prospects and seemingly different values. I am probably wrong,

© Springer Nature Switzerland AG 2019
G. Filler, R. Nagra, *Becoming a Successful Scholar*,
https://doi.org/10.1007/978-3-030-24448-4_1

but I do detect a sense of entitlement among them. They were the "chosen ones," the "future"; they could choose jobs more easily, as there was much less competition.

Generation Y (also known as Millennials) represents the children of the baby boomers, born approximately between 1985 and 2005. They are quite different from their parents, as they generally grew up with a lot of exposure to communications, media, and digital technologies. However, in terms of competitiveness in school, postgraduate education and competition in the job market conditions are similar. Finding a dream job may be equally challenging as it was for boomers some 35 years earlier. Moreover, jobs are being abolished and replaced by computers or robots. The cutthroat atmosphere for both acceptance into the training programs and for employment is indeed exacerbating (Fig. 1.1).

Why am I elaborating on this? I am such a boomer. Similar to what you as a Generation Y member experience today, the competition was fierce. I was born in West Germany, during the years when the highest birth rates over the past seven decades were recorded. In the early 1960s, the birth rate in West Germany was 1.4 million births per year, about twice as high as in 2010. For a developed country of 60 million, this was a lot. Everything was a competition, similar to what you are probably experiencing today. Even just getting me into daycare must have been a nightmare for my parents.

Germany has a three-tier school system: *Hauptschule*, *Realschule*, or *Gymnasium*. Back then, there had to be a decision about which tier of the school system you would be allowed to enter as early as grade 5. While today there are ways to cross from one tier to another, back in the 1960s, it was close to impossible. Only pupils who graduated from the *Gymnasium* were able to go to university: the gateway to higher education and high-paying jobs. Everyone and anywhere, you were receiving the same message: Be the best, be productive, be successful, and be better than the competition! This message was not as strong for the Generation X members; however, it happened all over again for the Millennials.

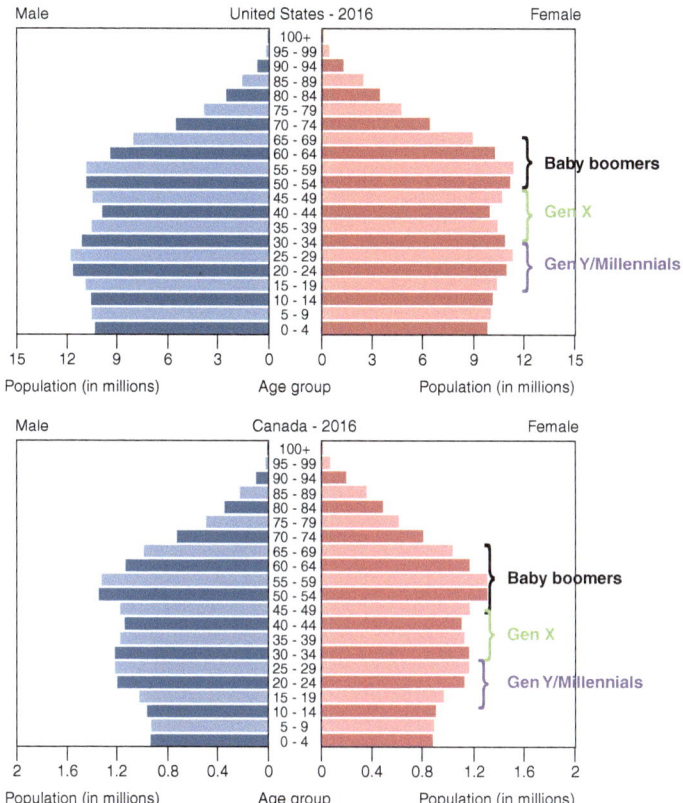

FIGURE 1.1 Population graphs of the United States and Canada

While I see this all from a distance after a successful career, back in the 1970s and 1980s, this threat was genuine, as it may be for many of you. I was 14 and a very sick child when I decided that I wanted to become a pediatrician, as my doctor had been a great inspiration. To get into medical school, I needed to have an "Abitur," the "high school diploma" for the third tier of the German school system, the Gymnasium.

I did not just have to get in the Gymnasium and pass. I had to be in the top 1% of Gymnasium graduates to get into medical school. At that time, the German universities relied on a system called "numerus clausus," which mostly meant you could only get into medical school with a 97% or higher average. It may sound unreal to some Generation Xers, but for us baby boomers, and likely for many Millennials, this was – or is – a very undeniable reality.

To further improve my fluency in English, I wanted to study the last year of high school in the United States of America. I applied to "Youth for Understanding" (an organization out Ann Arbor, Michigan, USA), which taught troubled youth democracy after World War II. At the time when I applied (1975), few Germans came to the USA. However, I matched to a wonderful family in Phoenix, Arizona, and I departed for my first year away from home when I was barely 17 years of age. I encourage young people to consider going a year abroad and getting out of their comfort zone. This may be unthinkable for many Millennials but may open up the door for many opportunities that may otherwise be missed.

The most incredible thing happened to me while still in Germany when I attended the preparation course for this year in Bonn, Germany. The instructor transformed my life. I was what the Millennials call a "geek" or "nerd," deprived of social relationships, with few friends, and entirely focused on being the top 1% that made it to medical school.

What the instructor taught me is that we are all assigned roles in life by our peers, parents, siblings, classmates, etc. Their expectations and opinions of you make it incredibly difficult for you to change your role. However, when you come to a new country where nobody knows you, you are like an unwritten book. You can assume any role you like.

I did just that. I wanted to be a socially responsible person. I was elected into the student council. This transformed my life and inspired me to assume leadership positions throughout my career. Not everyone will have opportunities like this. However, beginning at that time and throughout my career, I learned that certain behaviors would be extremely beneficial for success. This book is about these behaviors. Some may be quite surprising. It is not luck but *the return on luck* that determines your success. It is not the daring big project that determines your success but rather small and expendable projects that accumulate to high-impact projects. Binge working does not lead to success. Instead, consistency and regular daily work will serve as a critical enabler. Your mind will deceive you: if it perceives a less than 70% likelihood for success, you will procrastinate and not start the project. This is why it is important to divide your task into small little portions and schedule them into short, 45–60-minute assignments. Exercise fanatic discipline. You will not only get the work done on time but will always be ahead of schedule. Do the most challenging work or assignment first thing in the morning: the result will be an incredible boost in productivity.

This book begins with a chapter about why we should communicate our learnings. It will then expand on the mindset. You can increase your IQ, and a positive mindset will transform your productivity. Three behaviors that I shamelessly stolen from Jim Collins' and Morten T. Hansen's book, *Great by Choice*, are the cornerstones for your performance: fanatic discipline, productive paranoia, and empirical creativity. While the book *Great by Choice* deals with behaviors for companies that are successful in times of high change and considerable uncertainty, these behaviors can also be applied to individuals. I will explain what I mean by this in great detail.

This book is intended as a toolkit for young aspiring professionals that are required to deliver excellence. While this book is mostly designed for Generation Y/Millennials, it may also be of benefit for Generation X members. Each of the behaviors will pave the way to your success. Enjoy the reading and provide feedback.

London, Ontario. December 2018.

Chapter 2
Why Should We Publish?

What is not communicated does not exist!

The early humans (*homo* genus) stem back to the Paleolithic era. The age of speciation of *Homo sapiens* out of the ancestral *Homo erectus* (who roamed the world for over two million years) is estimated to have taken place between roughly 300,000 and 200,000 years ago. However, there was continued admixture from archaic human species until as late as 30,000 years ago. 200,000 years ago, there were many contemporary *Hominidae* like the Australopithecus. The reign of *Homo sapiens*, however, did not occur until about 100,000 to 70,000 years ago [1]. The evolution of the human intelligence is closely tied to the evolution of the human brain and to the origin of language.

Now, imagine yourself in the Stone Age. Young people learned from their peers through an apprenticeship. Elders taught their offspring techniques that they had learned from their elders. In spite of the slow accumulation of knowledge, some Stone Age cultures accomplished incredible achievements. For instance, Malta has been host to several ancient cultures and is home to some of the oldest free-standing structures in the world. Malta has a rich prehistoric history; however, what we know about it and their people is very limited. This old population represents one of the oldest polished

© Springer Nature Switzerland AG 2019
G. Filler, R. Nagra, *Becoming a Successful Scholar*,
https://doi.org/10.1007/978-3-030-24448-4_2

Stone Age cultures, and their historical remains form an incredible testimony of their highly developed culture preceding any written communication.

One such example is the Skorba Temple, which is believed to be built at 5200 BC. One of the most well-known megalithic sites in Malta is probably the Hypogeum of Hal-Saflieni, a carved-out underground complex from which the remains of 7000 human skeletons were found.

The hypogeum (hypogeum II, Fig. 2.1) offers a unique insight into the mind of the Maltese temple builders and reinforces the image of a culture valuing rituals of life and death.

Unfortunately, we know nothing about them. It is evident that the creators of these incredible relics had "Level 5 ambition" – a concept to be later discussed – as you will have. However, all of their skills and learnings have been lost because they had no written communication that could withstand time. We have to piecemeal their history together through archaeological techniques. The explosion of knowledge built on the cumulative experiences of our forefathers only happened after the introduction of written communication.

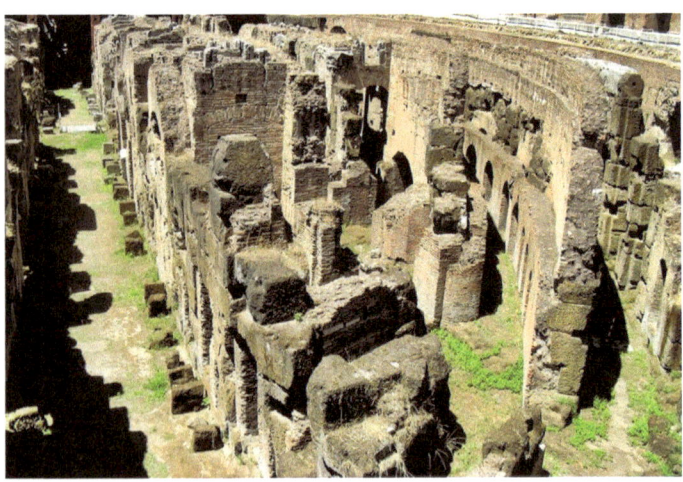

FIGURE 2.1 The hypogeum of Hal-Saflieni, Malta

When you visit these remains in Malta, a tour guide will ask you to make up a story, *any* story, about the statues. As you look at a figure, they will tell you that this was an important person. They will challenge you to invent a story about this person, as we know nothing about them, and your account might as well be the truth.

The key is written communication. In 3000 BC, Sumerians invented writing on clay tablets. About 500 years later, Egyptians invented hieroglyphics and papyrus. In China, animal bones with Chinese pictograms were discovered from around 1500 BC. In the new world, Aztecs used beaten bark to paint information on.

The year 600 BC marks the Greek development of parchment. It was made of sheepskin, which was stretched and soaked in lime for 2 weeks to preserve it, thin it, and harden it. Later, around the year 105 AD, more economical paper was produced from a variety of materials.

The first printing press was invented in the year 593 AD in China. In the following three centuries, papermaking techniques went over to Korea and Japan and later to the Middle East. The knowledge of how to make paper came to Europe in the year 1100 AD. The year 1238 AD marks the year European paper mills began being produced in Spain. Johannes Gutenberg, a German who died on February 3, 1468, invented the moveable printing press (Fig. 2.2).

The printing press was a dramatic improvement to earlier printing methods where the medium was brushed or rubbed to achieve printing. This technique was the critical enabler for book printing, which marks the explosion of education and knowledge in Europe. In 1476, a press was set up in Westminster, England, which enabled mass printing.

Further refinement of communication to the masses occurred with the development of the Internet (Fig. 2.3). Book printing and the Internet were the most influential tools for mass education and the explosion of knowledge. The Internet provided the entire world with access to cumulative information gathered by previous generations, which is currently expanding at an exponential rate.

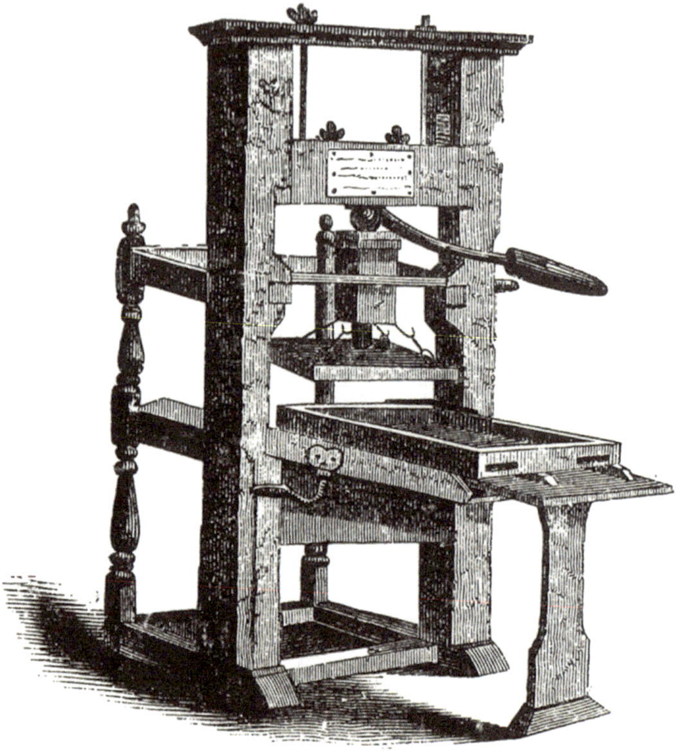

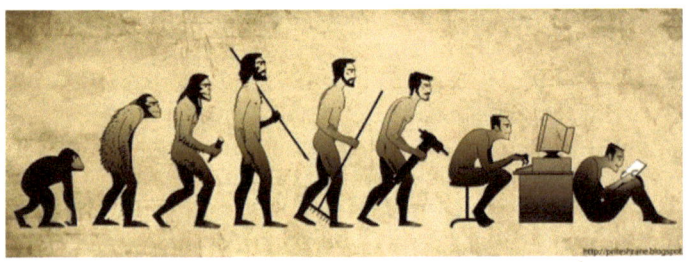

FIGURE 2.2 Gutenberg printing press

FIGURE 2.3 The evolution and "de-evolution" of man. Clearly, this is meant to be funny, but the Internet may actually be the key enabler for education of the entire world

Why am I dwelling on the importance of written communication? Our evolution from apprentice-type learning from one generation to the next to modern society is first and foremost the product of the explosion of communicated knowledge. Unfortunately, a lot of really good learnings have been lost because they have not been communicated.

You can be the world's best doctor or the world's best biochemist, but if you don't communicate your learnings, they will not exist after your demise. I will ask you, the reader, to forgive me for using predominantly medical examples only because I am a physician. Undoubtedly, similar cases can be found for any science or field of investigation. Written communication forms the most crucial tool for communication of knowledge.

What is not written does not exist!

Therefore, the question is never "Why should I publish?" but rather "Why should I NOT publish?" We are fortunate that we have all these tools at the tip of our fingers. We must use them to contribute to the cumulative knowledge of humanity.

Reference

1. Nichols J. The origin and dispersal of languages: linguistic evidence. In: Jablonski N, Aiello LC, editors. The origin and diversification of language. (Memoirs of the California Academy of Sciences, 24). San Francisco: California Academy of Sciences; 1998. p. 127–70.

Chapter 3
Lack of Evidence-Based Guidance

If we have a teachable moment, it should be shared
You can be the world's best physician, but if it is not communicated, it does not exist!
Correlation does NOT imply causation!

Written information forms the basis of today's understanding of what we think is right and true. We all learn about "evidence-based medicine" and how we should apply evidence for medical decision-making. However, the British Medical Journal reckons that 50% of medical treatments aren't proven, while 5% are actually harmful but are still being used [1]. Even among treatments that are supported with good evidence, only 15% were rated as beneficial, 22% as likely to be beneficial, 7% partially beneficial and partially harmful, 5% unlikely to be beneficial, 4% likely to be ineffective or even harmful, and the remaining 47% of treatment has an unknown effect [2].

To say that we have to use evidence for medical decision-making would leave the provider in a difficult situation. Not only is the available evidence often not good, but there are many situations where we have no evidence at all.

We have to provide treatment. The research community has been commendably diligent. Unfortunately, for rare diseases, there is rarely enough patient volume, even in an entire country, to perform a randomized control trial, the gold standard for clinical research. Randomized control trials also

© Springer Nature Switzerland AG 2019
G. Filler, R. Nagra, *Becoming a Successful Scholar*,
https://doi.org/10.1007/978-3-030-24448-4_3

often fail to prove that a particular treatment is useful, as they are underpowered, or were never designed as a superiority trial, but rather as a non-inferiority trial. Whereas a superiority trial aims at finding a better therapy, a noninferiority trial tests whether a new experimental treatment is not unacceptably less efficient than an active control treatment already in use. There are other levels of evidence which may be much more beneficial, such as case series or even $n = 1$ studies. These provide incredible learnings. However, in the current teaching, randomized control trials and meta-analyses of randomized control trials are considered the highest level of evidence.

Let me illustrate this with an example. In 2002, I met a 12-year-old girl who was born with chronic constipation and plagued with recurrent infection and persistent fatigue. She also did not tolerate changes in posture well and responded with a very high heart rate (tachycardia). This unfortunate girl and her parents started on what would prove to be an exhaustingly long quest for answers. At the time of referral, she had already been seen by more than a dozen specialists and subspecialists, had undergone a number of tests (including neurophysiological testing), and still did not have a precise diagnosis. The proposed solutions were quite outrageous. For instance, a gastroenterologist suggested she undergo a bowel resection, which her parents (fortunately) refused. They believed there was a root cause to all of her suffering and were determined to find it.

Without going into too many details, the patient was eventually diagnosed with Ehlers-Danlos syndrome-associated autonomic dysfunction and cortisol deficiency. Unfortunately, it took 6 more years and referrals to two physicians, Dr. Peter Rowe (Johns Hopkins) and Dr. Blair Grubb (Toledo, both in the United States), before a final unifying diagnosis was made. It is not uncommon for Ehlers-Danlos syndrome to be associated with autonomic dysfunction [3] nor is the gastrointestinal manifestations [4]. However, while we eventually had a diagnosis, we had to provide treatment and help this unfortunate young lady with her predicament.

At this point, the drug pyridostigmine had been investigated for off-label use in adult postural orthostatic tachycardia syndrome (POTS) patients. POTS is a condition that affects circulation (blood flow). POTS is a form of orthostatic intolerance, the development of symptoms that come on when standing up from a reclining position and that may be relieved by sitting or lying back down. The patient clearly showed features of this and was likely to respond to pyridostigmine, but no dosing recommendations existed for children, and the drug disposition (pharmacokinetics) of the drug had not been studied. To facilitate the trial of this treatment, we, therefore, developed a test for pharmacokinetic monitoring. We used a newly developed semiautomated and specific high-performance liquid chromatography with tandem mass spectrometry assay, which is a precision method for the measurement of the drug level in the blood and established normal pharmacokinetics for children with myasthenia gravis. We then applied the learnings from those tests to the young patient [5]. We also demonstrated its efficacy in our patient. A dose of 60 mg resulted in a substantial decrease in the initial tachycardia response to upward tilt that persisted in the plateau phase. To accommodate the rapid metabolism during childhood, the patient received three doses over the day and walked away with a substantial improvement in her quality of life.

Today, at the age of 28, our patient is unrecognizable from the frail little girl that could barely walk into my office many years ago. After completing a Masters and Ph.D. in Physics, she is now working as a postdoc at a major American university. With the aid of compression stockings and a compression suit, she was able to successfully travel to present her Ph.D. research around the globe. She regularly walks over 2 km per day, thanks to physiotherapy and custom orthotics – a huge improvement from the pain that exercise used to cause her.

All of this would have been impossible without this family's determination on their long search for answers. We will talk about perseverance later. Unfortunately, not all families are so resourceful. Autonomic dysfunction is understudied and under-taught. Centers for autonomic dysfunction are just emerging now and only for adult patients [6]. Academic health sciences centers are the last frontier for undiagnosed diseases, the last hope for patients that have often been through so much despair. We are fortunate to work in a country where the governments of the provinces acknowledge the need for such research and allow and remunerate for a proportion of scholarly activities to help patients like ours. Thus, it is our duty to our patients to utilize all resources at our disposal for diagnosis and treatment. We must not accept the failure to diagnose patients with rare diseases. Once we have diagnosed, we must not let a lack of tested treatment options resign us to inaction. We must not back away from these challenges, but instead, take the time as doctors to search for the answers our patients need. The rewards for doing so, as this patient has taught us, can be incredible.

Not only do we need more evidence, but we also have to be very mindful about what gets presented to us as evidence. Sometimes humanity gets it wrong. For instance, when analyzing the Framingham data, (a large epidemiological study in the United States), researchers found that total cholesterol level was significantly associated with the risk of coronary heart disease. While the researchers adjusted for other risk factors, by adding the various lipid levels in the blood of a patient, namely, the "bad" low-density lipoprotein (LDL) cholesterol and the "good" high-density lipoprotein (HDL) cholesterol, they considerably improved the prediction of risk [7]. An important finding of the North American population studied in the Framingham study was the fact that they ate significantly more fat than control cohorts. This was inferred as causality. This association has led to considerable unfavorable changes in the dietary habits of North America. The food industry discovered that the highly addictive fat in the food could be replaced with even more addictive sugars. There was never any actual proof that dietary fat affects the bad cholesterol LDL. It was not until much later that the association of a carbohydrate-rich diet, especially with high-fructose corn starch syrup, is more responsible for the formation of dangerous cholesterol fractions. Nowadays it is almost impossible to get high fat from cottage cheese or yogurt, but instead, we are exposed to much more perilous sugar supplements and high salt content. Notably, the explosion of the obesity pandemic coincided with these changes in food processing. The flooding of the food market with low cholesterol products contributed to an increase in the risk of cardiovascular morbidity and mortality, contrary to what the Framingham study suggested. Communicating our findings is exponentially essential, but it is also necessary to be critical of the claims studies make.

Cholesterol is not just merely bad. We require it in our diet. Even the so-called bad cholesterol, the LDL, is not generally harmful. LDL delivers fat molecules to the cells. Yes, it can drive the progression of atherosclerosis, but only if they become oxidized within the walls of arteries. Only some specific subfractions of LDL cholesterol, small-dense LDL (sd-LDL), and glycated LDL (g-LDL) are the dangerous fractions of the LDL.

Let us look at this in more detail. We give millions of patients statins, a class of medications which are proven to lower LDL cholesterol. However, an improvement in survival was never demonstrated, as the actual dangerous subgroup of sd-LDLs – a predictor of diseases such as cardiovascular morbidity – are unaffected. This is why we need more research.

When you order a lipid profile, the lab does not even measure LDL cholesterol. Instead, LDL is calculated using the Friedewald equation, which significantly was created back in 1972, is only reliable in specific cases, and cannot even be used in many patients due to the presence of specific biomolecules in their vasculature.

However, we have placed so much emphasis on the use of statins for the treatment of dyslipidemias, which exists outside of just the typical familial hypercholesterolemia and is prevalent in chronic kidney disease. In chronic kidney disease, the LDL lipids may remain normal, but regardless statins have been widely used in these patients while never having been proven to alter cardiovascular outcomes. In earlier small studies, it was suggested that statins might slow the progression of chronic kidney disease, but on the contrary, more extensive trials and more recent meta-analyses indicate they do not work at all, and their use is no longer recommended. Researchers who have worked vigorously to study the medicines we use and who have refused to accept outdated, while perhaps familiar, treatment methods have allowed for the production of different lipid-lowering substances. For instance, fibrates are the only class of lipid-lowering medications that affect sd-LDL [8].

So why do we dwell on this? There is constant progress, and we need to continue to dig for answers. We should strive to go by Sir Karl Popper's falsification theory.

For Popper, the growth of human knowledge proceeds from our problems and from our attempts to solve them. These attempts involve the formulation of theories which, if they are to explain anomalies which exist concerning earlier theories, must go beyond existing knowledge and therefore require a leap of the imagination. Curiosity and ingenuity are constantly needed for the progression of philosophy and science. We can always continue to acquire more knowledge, which in turn can only help improve current treatment methods and available medicine.

For this reason, Popper places particular emphasis on the role played by the independent creative imagination in the formulation of a theory. The centrality and priority of problems in Popper's account of science are paramount, and it is this which leads him to characterize scientists as "problem-solvers." Further, since the scientist begins with problems rather than with observations or "bare facts," Popper argues that the only sound technique which is an integral part of scientific method is that of the deductive testing of theories, which are not themselves the product of any logical operation. In this deductive procedure, conclusions are inferred from a tentative hypothesis. These conclusions are then compared with one another and with other relevant statements to determine whether they falsify or corroborate the hypothesis.

Curiosity is key! Enthusiasm and inquiry foster the expansion and progression of theories. Such conclusions are not directly compared with the facts simply because there are no "pure" facts available. All observation statements are theory-laden and are as much a function of purely subjective factors (interests, expectations, wishes, etc.) as they are a function of what is objectively real.

In other words, we should constantly try to falsify the existing hypotheses to get closer to the truth. I'd like to argue that plausibly 80% of treatment provided by healthcare professionals is not evidence-based, and even evidence-based medicine is established upon the knowledge that requires constant updating and improvement. This is why you should remain curious and continue to ask questions. If you have learnings, you need to communicate them and contribute to the growth of evidence-based medicine; otherwise, your learnings will be lost afterward. Remember, you can be the world's best doctor and find the most riveting and ground-breaking information, but if it is not communicated, it essentially does not exist.

While the considerable emphasis on medical expert is essential, it is not enough. The medical expert competency is not currently accomplishing what it should. To achieve better health for your patients, much more has to be done. You cannot be *just* a medical expert. You have to be a *communicator,* a *collaborator,* a *leader,* a *health advocate,* a *scholar,* and a *professional* (Fig. 3.1).

When individuals venture out to purchase a car, it is rare that they do so without first educating themselves and conducting their research. It is unlikely and uncommon for a car sales associate to assume their consumers know nothing. It may even be the case that they know *more* than the salesman! To effectively convince us to make a purchase, the salesman need not present us with a list of facts and details about the car, but rather, needs to be attuned to our specific needs.

Similarly, as a physician, your patients will come to you with their knowledge and opinions regarding their needs. With the Internet at one's fingertips, patients or parents or children or patients can quickly accumulate a lot of insight into a condition or disease or may even know about new

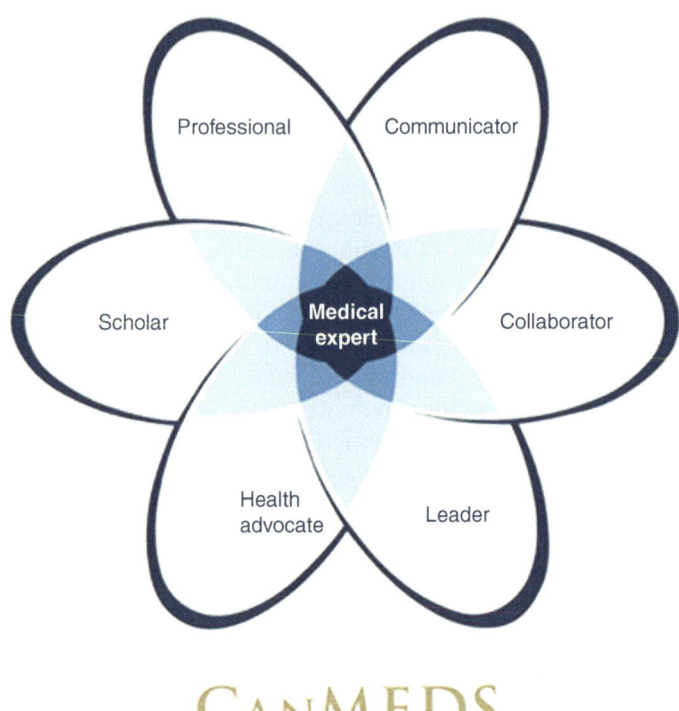

CanMEDS

FIGURE 3.1 The key core competencies of a physician as outlined by the Royal College of Physicians and Surgeons of Canada

medications or treatments before you do. We need to be prepared for that. Families also quickly find online resources. One mother of a child with a sporadic disorder quickly connected to both Canadian and US self-help interest groups for information and challenged me when I rounded the dose of the most crucial medication up. I worked it out to be 71 mg/kg, whereas the recommended dosing was 50–70 mg/kg. The mother was not satisfied until I lowered the dose below 70 mg/kg. Such action is likely to become the norm in the future. You will need to be able to back up all of your decisions, particularly when they are not entirely evidence-based, and the best way is to publish your learnings. In many fields, especially in the medical field, this is done through peer-reviewed papers in national or international journals.

Publishing papers and communicating your findings are essential for progress in the healthcare field. To assist patients with rare diseases, to debunk myths regarding our health, and to provide innovative treatment methods, ambitious individuals such as yourself are needed. We need to conduct research and communicate our findings in hopes of advancing the field of medical expertise.

In addition to progressing the healthcare field, there are also a lot of personal benefits to writing papers. For a start, writing a paper is an enjoyment. It is fun! Your employer may also oblige you; however, I do not think that this should be a reason to publish. Every paper that you publish also increases your likelihood of obtaining a grant. Not only that, but you may get a benefit or promotion, which ultimately translates into financial gain.

Now that we have thoroughly deciphered why we should publish in the first place, the next step is becoming familiar with the behaviors that will assist you in becoming a successful publishing scholar.

References

1. Cope J. The great debate. *Healthwriter.* 2007. p. 1–3.
2. Garrow JS. How much of orthodox medicine is evidence based? BMJ. 2007;335:951.
3. Celletti C, Camerota F, Castori M, et al. Orthostatic intolerance and postural orthostatic tachycardia syndrome in joint hypermobility syndrome/Ehlers-Danlos syndrome, hypermobility type: neurovegetative dysregulation or autonomic failure? Biomed Res Int. 2017;2017:9161865.
4. Nelson AD, Mouchli MA, Valentin N, et al. Ehlers-Danlos syndrome and gastrointestinal manifestations: a 20-year experience at Mayo Clinic. Neurogastroenterol Motil. 2015;27:1657–66.
5. Filler G, Gow RM, Nadarajah R, et al. Pharmacokinetics of pyridostigmine in a child with postural tachycardia syndrome. Pediatrics. 2006;118:e1563–e8.

6. UToday.   https://www.ucalgary.ca/utoday/issue/2015-10-22/first-autonomic-nervous-system-disorder-clinic-opens-calgary. (2015).
7. Castelli WP, et al. Lipids and risk of coronary heart disease. The Framingham Study. Ann Epidemiol. 1992;2(1–2):23–8.
8. Filippatos TD, et al. Safety considerations with fenofibrate/simvastatin combination. Expert Opin Drug Saf. 2015;14(9):1481–93.

Chapter 4
Fanatic Discipline

"Victory awaits him who has everything in order – luck people call it. Defeat is certain for him who has neglected to take the necessary precautions in time; this is called bad luck." Roald Amundsen

"Our luck in weather is preposterous… it is more than our share of ill fortune… how great may be the element of luck!" Robert Falcon Scott

A key enabler for your path to scholarly success is fanatic discipline, a skill which allows for your productivity to last beyond the shorter-lived inspiration that temporarily motivates and moves you. Why would we want to discipline ourselves? To answer that question, let us make a leap to the South Pole. I shamelessly confess that the comparison presented here is taken from Jim Collin's book, *Great By Choice*. However, as this insightful book is intended for aspiring business individuals and you may not have read it, I have decided to summarize the excellent metaphor described in order to explain the significance behind exercising fanatic discipline.

We are now in the year 1912. Two well-known gentlemen embarked on a race to the South Pole. They both had Level 5 Ambition: however, they could not be more different in their personalities (note the quotes at the beginning of this chapter). First, there was Roald Amundsen from Norway (1872–1928), who took 52 huskies, 5 men, and 3 tons of supplies with him on his expedition. Amundsen chose a slightly shorter

© Springer Nature Switzerland AG 2019

G. Filler, R. Nagra, *Becoming a Successful Scholar*,
https://doi.org/10.1007/978-3-030-24448-4_4

path, which included a tall mountain range. The second was Robert Falcon Scott (1868–1912), from Scotland. Scott did not bring any huskies, had 17 men with him, and 1 ton of supplies. He chose a very different route than Amundsen and decided to follow the same route on which he had previously been forced to return with his expedition incomplete. Currently, the Norwegian flag is waving over the South Pole, and we can all deduce the outcome of the story.

There is a behavior exercised by Amundsen that importantly illustrates the importance of fanatic discipline. Prior to the excursion, Amundsen determined 17 miles would be the safe distance within the red line of exhaustion. On December 12, 1911, Amundsen and his team had reached a point 45 miles from the South Pole. He had no idea of Scott's whereabouts, who was likely ahead. The weather had turned clear and calm, and sitting on the flat polar plateau, Amundsen got the benefit of having perfect ski and sled conditions. His team had journeyed more than 650 miles, and now everybody was very excited because they could reach the South Pole in 24 hours. What did Amundsen do?

He said, "over my dead body!" Amundsen had vouched to bring everyone home without a frozen toe and pledged not to cross his team's red line of exhaustion. He insisted on marching only the 17 miles and not any more. Nevertheless, he led his team to success, and even today, the South Pole bears the Norwegian flag. He also brought his team back to safety without a frozen toe, as promised.

What happened to Scott? He arrived much later. You can see the disappointment in his face in the Fig. 4.1 below.

Scott, if he weren't a naval officer, would have been a scientist. Possessed with Level 5 Ambition, he made his teammates collect geological samples, so that there would be something additionally extraordinary to bring home. He deemed the slate samples with fossils precious early on, even though their value was not recognized by the public until much later. However, to take this extra weight along was a risk due to the fact that they were already running low on supplies and the men were exhausted. On the way back, Petty

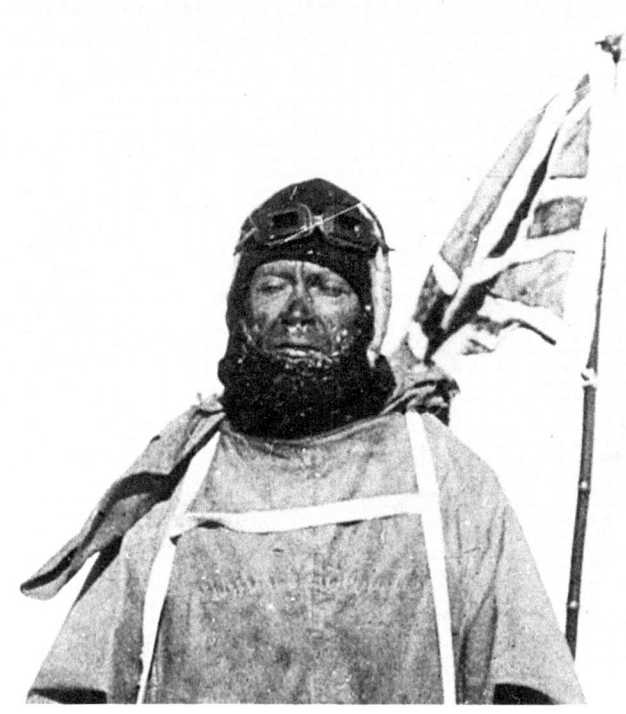

FIGURE 4.1 Imagine the devastation when your lifetime dream is destroyed as Robert Falcon Scott arrived at the South Pole only to find the Norwegian flag marking his defeat

Officer Edgar Evans calculated that there would be no hope for them to return based on the supplies left. Things got so bad that in the act of last resort, when the men camped, Evans stated he was going for a walk, but his real intent was to commit suicide in an attempt to improve the odds for the team. He died in February of 1912. Unfortunately, even with this heroic act, the rest of Scott's team died later, only 11 miles away from the base camp. They got caught in a 10-day snow storm and were forced to camp and stay in their tents: their last resting place. They had insufficient supplies and crossed the red line of exhaustion multiple times, deeming them for failure.

The bodies of Scott, Dr. Edward Wilson, and Lieutenant Bowers were eventually found in their tent by a search party in November 1912. At his time, Scott's mission was viewed as a heroic failure. The team did not execute the fanatic discipline that was necessary, and they crossed the red line of exhaustion in the process (see further down).

But was it all in vain? In the latter half of the twentieth century, Scott's status was re-examined. Alongside their bodies were several pounds of their precious geological samples and scientific notebooks. The team collected specimens from 2109 different animals. Of these, 401 were new to science [1]. They also collected rock samples, penguin eggs, and plant fossils. One of the most important discoveries was a fossilized fern-like plant which was known to grow in India, Africa, New Zealand, and Australia. It suggested that the climate 250 million years ago had been mild enough for trees to grow. Even more intriguing, the discovery, along with other evidence gathered by Scott's team, was a hint that Australia and Antarctica had in the distant past all been part of one "supercontinent." Researchers now call this landmass Gondwanaland. Gondwana was an ancient supercontinent that broke up about 180 million years ago. The continent eventually split into landmasses we recognize today: Africa, South America, Australia, Antarctica, the Indian subcontinent, and the Arabian Peninsula [2].

In real life, we should never cross the red line of exhaustion if we want to get anything done. If you're going to be a pediatrician, you need to read the *Nelson Textbook of Pediatrics*. Ideally, not once, or twice, but thrice. The latest addition has 3888 pages. On the very first day of your residency, you already know when you will have your final exam. Assuming that you have 880 working days from the beginning to end of pediatric residency, if you read the Nelson once, you would have to read 4.4 pages per day. I should point out that the 880 days do not include weekends, do not comprise statutory holidays, and account for any post-call days. If you're going to read the Nelson twice, you have to read 8.8 pages per day. If you want to read the Nelson thrice, you have to read 13.2 pages per day.

What does that mean? Assuming that one page has nothing except words, with an average font size of 10/12, one page should not take more than 3 minutes with full concentration. You can likely read 400 words per page, at a rate of 200 words per minute. Rarely is there a page in the Nelson without an illustration. This allows for the time calculated of 3 minutes for one page to include time for highlighting and writing notes. You can process 20 pages per hour. As such, you need to allow only 40 minutes every day during your residency to get through the 13.2 pages, a manageable task. You cannot read the Nelson in a month before the exam. However, you can spare 40 minutes every day to read 13.2 pages.

So, find your 17-mile march. Find your red line of exhaustion. Schedule the work. Put it into small little pieces that are manageable. Be mindful of your deceiving mind, which will procrastinate and prevent you from starting any project that seems too overwhelming. If your mind does not have an immediate perceived likelihood of success of at least 70%, it will suspend your will to commit to the plan. Rather than facing the 100-mile march all at once, focus on 17 miles at a time.

So, break things down. You can manage 40 minutes of learning every day (that is, every *work*day). Your mind will consider this a piece of cake. The regularity of your work will ensure that you go beyond your goal that you have set, by the sheer virtue of habitually doing it. You may find that you always end up ahead of schedule.

So how does this translate into being a scholar? If you procrastinate until that week of vacation to do all your research at once, you will not do it (because you need the vacation)! Again, your mind will not start anything that does not have at least a 70% likelihood of success. So instead, break your project down into small chunks that you can efficiently manage. For instance, allow 5 days, 1 hour each, for the literature review. Allow 1 day (1 hour), for the introduction. Rather than writing your methods with the rest of your paper, write the methods as you design your study and just cut and paste it afterward. Then write the results, perhaps broken down into three or four 1-hour sessions. For the discussion, break it down into four paragraphs:

1. A brief summary of the main results of the study (1 hour)
2. Explanation of the findings, comparison and contrast with other relevant findings in the literature (one or two paragraphs and 1 or 2 hours)
3. Limitations of the study (1 hour, one paragraph)
4. Conclusion and future directions in the area of the research (1 hour)

You will likely find that you need much less time to complete this discussion in comparison to the timeline outlined above if you focus and attend to the task at hand in small pieces.

Also, do one of the most challenging tasks of your day first thing in the morning. You will be amazed what that does to your day's success. Because you have mastered a hurdle first thing in the morning, your day will be much more productive. Procrastinating the hard things and pushing them aside until you face an insurmountable time pressure is the perfect recipe for misery.

Another good behavior to enhance your productivity is to consider several projects at different phases in parallel. It takes a long time to execute the process of a complete project: from the conception of an idea, to writing an ethics protocol, to getting it through ethics, applying for grant funding, assembling your research team, enrolling patients, entering the data, analyzing the data, summarizing the results for a presentation, and finally writing the manuscript is no quick and easy process. If you have half a dozen projects at different stages and you keep getting one coming to fruition at a time every month, you can publish a dozen papers a year. If you want to work just through one project at a time from A to Z, it may take you years to complete. So map things out. Complete short tasks regularly and in a disciplined manner. Be strategic. Consider using a project software. I use MeisterTask Version 1.2.11, which is platform independent, works on handheld devices and desktops, and it is free!

Also, be in what Stephen Covey calls Quadrant 2. All tasks can mainly be divided into categories of importance. If you make a four-quadrant table and label the columns as either *urgent* or *not urgent* and the rows as *important* or as *not important*, you end up with the quadrants below (Fig. 4.2). Quadrant 2

	Urgent	Not urgent
Important	**Quad I** **Activities** · Crisis · Pressing Problems · Deadline Driven **Results** · Stress · Brun-out · Crisis management · Always putting out fires	**Quad II** **Activities** · Prevention, capability improvement · Relationship building · Recognizing new opportunities · Planning, recreation **Results** · Vision, perspective · Balance · Discipline · Control · Few crisis
Not important	**Quad III** **Activities** · Interruptions, some callers · Some email, some reports · Some meetings · Proximate, pressing matters · Popular activities **Results** · Short term focus · Crisis management · Reputation – chameleon character · See goals/ plans as worthless · Feel victimized, out of control · Shallow or broken relationships	**Quad IV** **Activities** · Trivia, busy work · Some email · Personal social media · Some phone calls · Time wasters · Pleasant activities **Results** · Total irresponsibility · Fired from jobs · Dependent on others or institutions for basics

Figure 4.2 Stephen Covey's Four Quadrant Plan of Activities

would be *important*, but *not urgent*. Active people stay out of Quadrants 3 and 4 because regardless of whether they are critical or not, they are *not important*. Effective people also shrink Quadrant 1 down in size by spending more time in Quadrant 2 and getting important tasks done *before* they become *urgent*. Quadrant 2 is the heart of effective project management.

Activities that belong under Quadrant 2 are focused on prevention, capability, and improvement. They focus on relationship building. I will talk a lot about relationships later. Quadrant 2 enables you to recognize new opportunities. Examples of activities include planning and recreation. The rewards are sumptuous. You get vision and perspective, you achieve balance, you exercise discipline and control, and you avoid a crisis.

If you are always in Quadrant 1 (*urgent and important*), which is crisis management, pressing problems, and deadline driven, you face stress, burnout, are in a constant mode of crisis management, or are always putting out fires. It is a recipe for disaster.

Far worse is being in Quadrant 3 (*urgent and not important*). Activities include interruptions, some callers, some emails, some reports, and meetings. There is a sense of proximity, of pressing matters, and they include favorite activities; however, they are simply insignificant. They will absorb your short-term focus, and you end up having to utilize your crisis management skills for other activities that are important. The price may even be a damaged reputation. The goals and plans you develop are wasted on unimportant and therefore worthless things. You feel victimized and out of control. It may even affect your relationships and result in shallow or even broken relationships. Do not spend any time in Quadrant 3, and it is just not important.

Quadrant 4 (*not urgent and not important*) reflects trivia, busy work, computer games, some emails, personal social media like Instagram or Facebook, and time wasters such as phone calls from advertising agencies or telemarketers. If you engage in these activities, you may endanger your productivity and might end up getting fired from your job. By spending too much time here, in order to meet your deadlines, you will end up depending on others or the institution for assistance, which will inevitably jeopardize your reputation. It is just not worth spending any time in Quadrant 4. This may be unpopular, but you may want to consider deleting your LinkedIn, Facebook, or Instagram social media account.

Time management is of the essence. I warmly recommend *The 7 Habits of Highly Effective People* by Stephen Covey. In fact, incorporating the learnings from this book will be foundational to your scholarly success. His book is full of advice on taking control of your life, teamwork, self-renewal, mutual benefit, proactivity, and other paths to private and public success (Fig. 4.3).

Just in case you have not read this book, here is a summary of the main habits. By embracing these habits, you move from dependence to independence and eventually to interdependence. It is not the case that everything is due to personality traits, but it is a habit. Integrating habit into your workflow enables you. Utilize the power of habits. These are:

- *Be proactive:* Work from the center of your influence and continuously work to expand it. Do not sit and wait in a reactive mode, waiting for problems to happen before taking action. Anticipate what may go wrong in your experiments and consult before acting.
- *Begin with the end in mind:* Envision the future, and what you want it to look like, so you can work and plan toward it. To be effective, you need to understand how people make decisions and to act based on principles and constantly review your mission statement. Change your life to act and be proactive according to Habit 1. You are the investigator, the scientist, and the scholar. Grow but stay humble.
- *Put first things first:* Identify the critical roles that make a scholar and make time for each of them. Spend time doing what should absolutely go into your personal and research agenda, observing the balance between deliverables (i.e., papers) and the capacity to produce them.

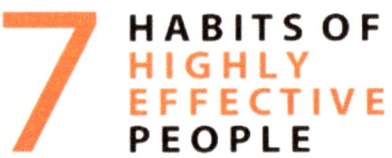

01. BE PROACTIVE

02. BEGIN WITH THE END IN MIND

03. PUT FIRST THINGS FIRST

04. THINK WIN - WIN

05. SEEK FIRST TO UNDERSTAND THEN TO BE UNDERSTOOD

06. SYNERGIZE

07. SHARPEN THE SAW

FIGURE 4.3 Stephen Covey's *The Seven Habits of Highly Effective People*. Especially important: sharpen the saw

- *Think win-win:* Seek contracts, work environments, and relationships that are *mutually* beneficial. In cases where a win-win deal cannot be achieved, do not be afraid to walk away from that deal. Valuing and respecting people by understanding a "win" for all is ultimately a better long-term solution as compared to have only one person having gotten their way.

- *Seek first to understand, then to be understood:* First seek to understand the other person, and only thereafter try to be understood. Putting oneself in the perspective of the other person and listening empathetically for feeling and meaning, rather than making assumptions and judgements, forms the basis for successful relationships that are required for being a successful scholar.

- *Synergize:* Through trustful communication, find ways to leverage individual differences to create a whole that is greater than the sum of the parts. Through mutual trust and understanding, one can often solve conflicts and find a better solution that would be obtained through either person's solution.

- *Sharpen the saw:* You cannot effectively cut a tree with a blunt saw, no matter how hard you try. You need to spend the time to sharpen the saw before beginning your work. This implies that you have your skills and tools ready and in pristine condition before you begin. For instance, you need to know your statistics program. You need to have a superior command of Excel. Word formatting issues should not slow you down. For your lifestyle, this means that you need to balance your resources, energy, and health to create a sustainable, long-term, effective career.

There is also an eighth habit, which is *to find your voice and inspire others to find theirs.* Taken together, fanatic discipline at your 17-mile march limit *within your red line of exhaustion* forms the foundational behavior for your successful career. The central idea of the eighth habit, which features a separate book, is the need for steady recovery and application of what Covey considers the "whole person paradigm," the unity of the physical, intellectual, emotional, and spiritual components of self. He states that denial of any of them reduces individuals to things and may result in many problems.

Now you might say that fanatic discipline is boring, that genius pours out, and that you have periods of incredible productivity. Well, let us examine this idea of fanatic discipline and effectiveness and productivity a bit more with the example of two famous composers, namely, Wolfgang Amadeus Mozart and Antonín Dvořák. We all know Mozart. His *Lacrimosa* from his *Requiem* or the second movement of his piano concerto Köchelverzeichnis (KV) 467 are two of the most soothing pieces of music that I can imagine. Wolfgang Amadeus Mozart was a prolific and influential composer of the classical era. Born in Salzburg on January 27, 1756, Mozart showed prodigious ability from his earliest childhood. When he was 8 years old, he wrote his first symphony (although some say his father mostly transcribed it). We all remember him for his genius. Early in his career, he had a steady job through the ruler of Salzburg, Prince Archbishop Hieronymus Colloredo, however, he grew increasingly discontented with Salzburg and tried hard to find a position elsewhere. He had a meager salary, 150 florins per year. Translating Mozart's income into today's dollar is a matter of educated guesswork because data on eighteenth-century prices and consumption habits is sparse. It seems that in the 1780s, one florin could roughly buy as much as $10 in 1989 (https://www.nytimes.com/1991/12/11/business/economic-scene-mozart-s-money-misunderstanding.html). In August 1777, Mozart resigned from his position at Salzburg and started his journey with visits to Augsburg, Mannheim, Paris, and Munich. His usual pattern began; he would burst out in bouts of productivity, sell his pieces, and live like a king for a few days which would rapidly fade, and then he was struggling until his next genius piece brought him new money. He aimed at working at the emperor and decided to move to Vienna as a freelance performer and composer. In Vienna, he often performed as a pianist and established himself as one of the best keyboard players of his time. In 1786 and 1787, he tried his success at the opera and wrote terrific pieces, such as "Die Entführung aus dem Serail," which was a great success. His income increased and fluctuated between 800 and 3800 Austrian Florins during his Vienna years or on average about $30,000 in today's money. The figure looks even better when one remembers that the purchasing power of the average wage in Mozart's Vienna was, at very most, one-seventh the average in America today. Mozart's income was thus enough to qualify him for Vienna's upper middle class. Nonetheless, his income was subject to substantial fluctuations based on his productivity. Toward the end of the decade, his circumstances worsened, his income shrunk, and money became very tight because of the Austro-Turkish war, which resulted in a dramatic decline of support for music from nobility.

Mozart moved to Alergrund, a suburb of Vienna, but instead of reducing his rental expenses, Mozart began to borrow money, most often from his friend Michael Puchberg. His output slowed, and some analysts suggest that he suffered from depression. Mozart's last year was, until his final illness struck, a time of high productivity when he composed some of his most admired work: the Magic Flute opera, the amazing clarinet concerto KV 622, and the motet Ave Verum Corpus (KV 618). This was also the year when he wrote the Requiem as mentioned above, which was mostly unfinished at the time of his early death at age 35. Mozart fell ill while in Prague for the September 6, 1791 premiere of his opera La Clemenza di Tito. His health deteriorated, and he became bedridden, suffering from swelling, pain, and vomiting. Mozart died in his home on December 5, 1791. The cause of death was recorded as "fever and rash," which even then were called symptoms, not a disease. Today, an epidemiological study of *The Annals of Internal Medicine* suggests that Mozart was a victim of an epidemic streptococcal infection. Deaths were routinely recorded in eighteenth-century Vienna, but physicians were not required to note a cause, which was usually provided by relatives or the clerk doing the paperwork. These records have survived, and the researchers used them to figure out patterns of death in the months surrounding Mozart's final illness – November and December 1791 and January 1792 – and compare them with the patterns in the same periods of the previous and following years. The scientists found 5011 deaths of people 18 and older over the 9 months. The most common causes were tuberculosis, malnutrition, edema (swelling of tissue under the skin), gastrointestinal disease, and cerebrovascular disease, the blood vessel disorder that leads to stroke. But in the winter of 1791–1792, edema was the only cause that showed an increased incidence among younger men compared with the other years, suggesting a small epidemic of infectious disease. Edema is also associated with certain chronic diseases of the kidneys and heart, but Mozart's sickness was sudden. In addition to the edema, Mozart had malaise, back pain, and a rash, all symptoms of streptococcal infection. Streptococcus is sometimes followed by an acute kidney disease called glomerulonephritis, which would explain the severe swelling [3]. He was buried in a common grave. What a sad death in complete poverty.

By contrast, Antonín Leopold Dvořák was a Czech composer, one of the first to achieve worldwide recognition. He lived from 1841 to 1904. He was the son of a butcher in Nelahozeves, now the Czech Republic. Similar to Mozart, his talent showed in early years, as he was an excellent violin player at as early as 6 years old. However, his career was undoubtedly much more pedestrian. In 1859 he started as a viola player in a private orchestra headed by Karel Komzák, where he stayed for a total of 11 years without composing. In 1865, Dvořák augmented his income with piano teaching and married one of his pupils, Anna Čermáková. He started composing music in 1870 at the age of 29 years, beginning with his opera Alfred. One year later, he resigned from his orchestra position to have more time for composing. The first successful piece was the hymnus *Die Erben des Weißen Berges* for choir and orchestra. His composing style could not be more different than that of Mozart. According to one biography, he composed 16 bars every day, no more, no less. In 1974, he received a regular stipend from the state for his compositions. It was no one less than Johannes Brahms who was on the committee and helped Dvořák by introducing his music to the publisher Fritz Simrock. He soon received more and more international invitations. In September of 1892, he accepted an offer to become the director of the *National Conservatory of Music* in New York. His annual salary was $15,000, which would reflect $415,447.25 in 2018 [4]. You may not be so familiar with his music, but I am confident that you recognize the *New World Symphony* [5]. It is hard to believe that this masterpiece was written in bouts of 16 bars, but when you look at the score, you can appreciate it. His contract was actually extended, but instead, he decided to return to his home in Europe in Bohemia in 1985. He considered relocation to Vienna, where he was also offered a lucrative position at the conservatory but decided against it. His fortune from work in the United States enabled him to buy a huge estate at the Kateňinská in Prague Neustadt, which he named "Villa America." Today, it houses the Dvořák Museum. There he continued to compose until his passing. He died on May 1, 1904, from a stroke. Thousands accompanied his funeral, and he was buried in the famous Vyšehrad Cemetery, where the most famous Czech personalities found the final resting place. He left many unfinished pieces with – you guessed it – 16 bar components.

Now I am asking you, the reader, if you would rather live Mozart's or Dvořák's life? True genius like Mozart is only given to very few in our world, yet fanatic discipline can give you genuinely exceptional results like the *New World Symphony* by Dvořák. When I am down, I listen to the Largo, the second movement, which is one of the most beautiful slow movements in the classical music, produced through the consistent and continuous efforts of Dvořák.

References

1. http://www.bbc.com/news/science-environment-16530953.
2. https://www.livescience.com/37285-gondwana.html.
3. https://www.nytimes.com/2009/08/18/health/18mozart.html.
4. http://www.in2013dollars.com/1892-dollars-in-2018?amount=15000.
5. https://www.youtube.com/watch?v=HClX2s8A9IE.

Chapter 5
Empirical Creativity

In *Great by Choice*, Collins and Hansen observe (Fig. 5.1):

> The 10xers (the highly resilient companies) were much more likely to fire calibrated cannonballs, while the comparison cases had uncalibrated cannonballs flying all over the place (the 10x cases had a 69 percent calibration rate on cannonballs versus 22 percent for the comparisons). Whether fired by the 10x case or the comparison case, calibrated cannonballs had a success rate nearly four times higher than uncalibrated cannonballs, 88 percent to 23 percent. (p. 74)

What do they mean by that and what does productivity have to do with cannon balls?

For centuries, the domination of the world by the colonial powers such as the British Empire was made possible because of the supremacy of the naval fleet. Cannonballs were of pivotal importance, as they provided superior firepower and caused devastating destruction even from far ashore. Initially, one cannonball was fired at a time, but later multiple cannonballs were fired at once to maximize the damage on the opposing ship. Especially during World War II, broadside ships were used to eliminate the opponent on the first strike. However, the firing of their canons caused a massive surge of smoke to rise and obstruct the view of the soldiers, making it immensely difficult to aim at their enemies accurately. Blindly shooting often rapidly resulted in exhaustion of their firepower supply and being left with no defenses. It was necessary

© Springer Nature Switzerland AG 2019   39
G. Filler, R. Nagra, *Becoming a Successful Scholar*,
https://doi.org/10.1007/978-3-030-24448-4_5

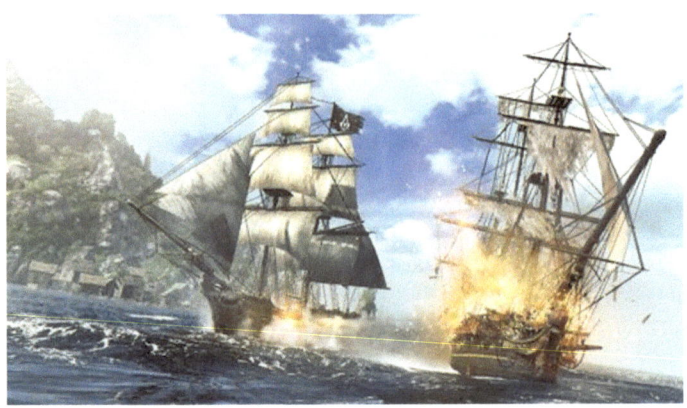

FIGURE 5.1 Powder dust makes aiming impossible during naval warfare

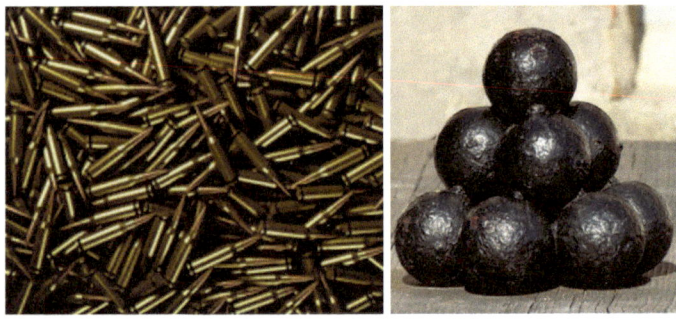

FIGURE 5.2 Whereas a rather large number of bullets (more expendable resource) could be brought along, the volume and weight of the cannon balls limited the amounts loaded onto the ship

for them to adopt a new method in order to have any hope of being victorious. This was especially true before targeting devices such as radar were invented.

Consider the following two pictures (Fig. 5.2):

Yes, the cannonballs may be more impactful, more potent, but the amount of gunpowder required to shoot one cannonball is enormous, especially in comparison to the amount needed to fire a single bullet. A ship could also carry only a

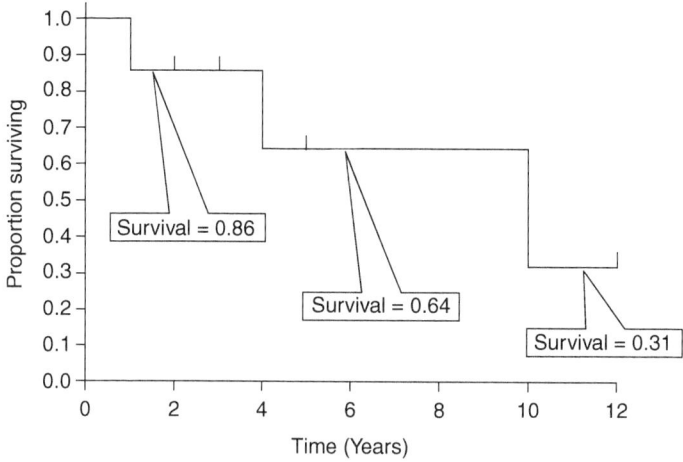

FIGURE 5.3 Kaplan-Meier plot – indicating chances of survival

limited supply of the very heavy cannonballs. What happens if you use up all your ammunition and at the same time haven't hit your target a single time? (Fig. 5.3)

With every cannonball shot, the teams would diminish their chances of survival by drastically reducing the number of resources they had, similar to the stepladder-like decline seen on this Kaplan-Meier plot. With every cannonball in the water, the survivorship of the crewmates diminished significantly. They needed to adopt a new method to ensure that every cannonball would find its target: firing *bullets and then cannonballs* were the pivotal moment for these soldiers. Consider the difference in the amount of resources required when firing a bullet rather than a cannon. If you miss your target, no problem! Readjust your aim by 10 degrees, load your bullet, and try again. If the bullet still splashes into the water, you still have a large amount of firepower available. Readjust your aim again before firing the next bullet by 10 degrees or so and continue to do so until the bullet hits the other ship. Only then is it time for the cannonball, when your cannon can undoubtedly hit its bullseye!

Think of your research resources as the sum of the cannon-balls, gunpowder, cannons, rifles, bullets, etc. One cannonball is a lot less expendable than a bullet. The important takeaway from this is that expendable resources – while not necessarily having an enormous, explosive impact – can be used for proof of concept (PoC) or proof of principle (PoP) without exhausting your grants. PoC is a realization of a particular method or idea in order to demonstrate its feasibility or a demonstration in principle with the aim of verifying that some concept or theory has practical potential. PoC is usually small and may or may not be complete. PoP studies, on the other hand, reflect an early stage of clinical drug development when a compound has shown potential in animal models and initial safety testing. These small-scale studies are designed to detect a signal that the drug is active on a pathophysiologically relevant mechanism, as well as preliminary evidence of efficacy in a clinically relevant endpoint. Sponsors use these studies to estimate whether their compound might have clinically significant efficacy in other diseases states. It is better to perform several pilot studies with more expendable resources rather than "firing a broadside." Burning your entire grant within the first few assaults in battle, you will surely lose the war, and it may cost you your career.

Resources are hardly available in an unlimited manner unless you are playing a virtual reality game. In video games, if you use all of your character's energy points or lives, you can easily fall back on cheat codes you find on the Internet to replenish your resources, try the level again (as many times as you like), and beat the game. If life were as simple as video games, you would not need to have single care of how hastily or impulsively you use your resources. Firing as many can-nonballs as you want would be completely fine. Unfortunately, the reality is not that effortless. It is exceedingly hard even to get a grant and almost impossible without pilot data and pilot projects. For instance, you may have to perform an expensive assay for your main hypothesis, but you do not know if it will provide you with the results that you need. Let us assume you have a grant over $40,000. Rather than testing all of your blood samples at once, you could choose to pilot this by mea-suring the expensive test in a small subset first to see if the results are supporting your hypothesis. Let us assume your assay is $150/sample. Instead of having paid $30,000 or 75% of your grant money on all 200 samples, you would have only spent $3000 on the 20 samples. If the assay did not work, you can always *zoom out* (a concept that will be discussed later) and consider a different approach without having much of your grant funding already spent. If you extinguish all your resources rapidly and do not hit your bullseye, you are left without the means to complete your projects.

A successful scholar by choice (you), will not foolishly attempt to fire all their large cannonballs, or projects, at once unless they want to end up putting everything they have worked toward at risk by aggregating all their resources into one large idea. Low-risk and low-investment opportunities that can validate your hypotheses and allow you to fine-tune your line of fire will be what enables you to get from good, to better, and to your best scholarly work. Small, methodological projects, although they may not be your primary goal, are *essential.* By evaluating and legitimizing your small, proven ideas, you can calibrate your cannonballs to get well-deserved recognition and the actual outcome desired with your cannonball or your mind-blowing project. Nothing great can be produced without foundation. Smaller projects and studies will provide you with the empirical evidence that will support your more extensive, more robust research and allow you to strive toward your objective confidently

Let us illustrate this with some examples. The National Institutes of Health (NIH) funded a large and expensive study for children with chronic kidney disease entitled the Chronic Kidney Disease in Children or CKiD study, which started in 2006. This study was a prospective cohort study of children aged 6 months to 16 years with mild to moderately impaired kidney function. The primary goals of CKiD are to:

1. Determine the risk factors for the decline in renal function
2. Define how progressive decline in renal function impacts the biomarkers of risk factors for cardiovascular disease, neurocognitive function and behavior, and growth failure and its associated morbidity.

Two clinical coordinating centers (located at Children's Hospital of Philadelphia and Children's Mercy Hospital in Kansas City), a central biochemistry laboratory (at the University of Rochester), and a data coordinating center (at Johns Hopkins School of Public Health) formed a cooperative agreement to conduct the CKiD study.

While not participating in the study because of a lack of resources in our center, I followed this ambitious project very carefully. I have been interested in trace elements. Essentially, the nephrologist needs to adjust any substance that accumulates or gets lost in CKD. It has always baffled me that we measure every electrolyte but ignore zinc, selenium, and other trace elements.

In adult dialysis patients, there is evidence for three different behaviors of trace elements. Some get lost, such as selenium, zinc, and manganese. Others are unaffected, and some renally excreted trace elements accumulate such as lead, molybdenum, chromium, vanadium, possibly cobalt, and others. Trace elements have rarely been studied in children with CKD, and almost nothing is known regarding their natural progression during worsening renal failure. For many of these trace elements, we do not even have reference intervals in children.

The best way to test trace elements over time is actually the hair. I knew from my friends who were participating in the CKiD trial that hair samples were collected at the beginning of the study and yearly intervals, and on top of this, the investigators had done nothing at all with the hair samples since the inception of the study.

So, I boldly went ahead and applied for the use of those hair samples. The study was rejected with the hint that I would be embarking on a total fishing expedition and the valuable resources being utilized would not guarantee new valuable knowledge. There was just a lack of studies of trace elements in children and adolescents with CKD.

In particular, the reviewers said that there is a "lack of normative data for many of the elements you propose." Further, there is a total "lack of preliminary data." One cannot simply project the results from adults with end-stage renal disease on to children with CKD, as trace element concentrations are age-dependent. Finally, they said "there's limited data to support the hypothesis," which was that selenium, zinc, and manganese deficiency would progressively worsen with CKD, whereas chromium, vanadium, molybdenum, cobalt, and lead would gradually accumulate.

So, I went ahead and fired bullets! The first study was a simple cross-sectional study of children with CKD in our center for elevated lead levels. Surprisingly, we found a very high prevalence of elevated lead levels in these patients. The second step was an in-depth review for the journal *Pediatric Nephrology* on the subject. After that, I tagged on an ancillary study to a trial on zinc supplementation in CKD patients, which I was undertaking with my friend Vladimir Belostotsky, from Hamilton. We were mainly interested if zinc supplementation would lower fibrosis growth factor 23 and normalize zinc deficiency. I sought funding for an ancillary study of this trial and measured first molybdenum in these patients and found an impressive exponential rise in the plasma of these patients with worsening GFR. My bullets were getting closer and closer to the target, and these small lower-risk projects allowed me to accumulate the support I needed to justify loading up my cannonball and utilizing greater resources (Fig. 5.4).

We subsequently published this in the Journal of *Clinical Nephrology*. Then we looked at vanadium and chromium. We found exactly the same pattern. This was published in *BMJ Open*. Both vanadium and chromium are highly toxic when in excess in the body. We also found that the concentration of these two trace elements was dependent on the drinking water and showed dramatic variation across the province of Ontario (Fig. 5.5).

Currently, we are studying cobalt, which is particularly interesting because it can cause cardiomyopathy, which is a common cause of death in children and young adults with end-stage kidney disease. And of course, we found a high prevalence of high cobalt levels in these patients. So now

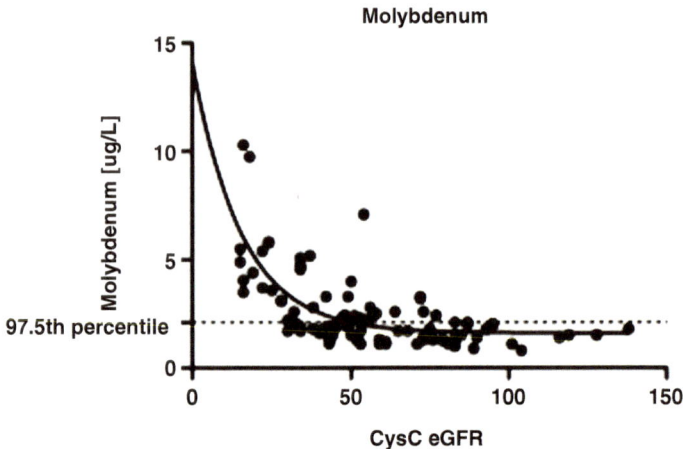

FIGURE 5.4 A figure from the ancillary study: the relationship between the estimated glomerular filtration rate based on serum cystatin C concentration (CysC eGFR) and the molybdenum level in plasma. It showed an exponential accumulation with lower eGFR, since this trace element is renally eliminated

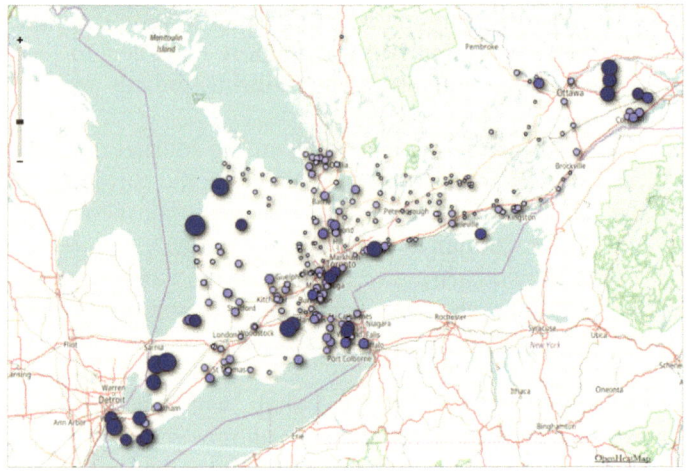

FIGURE 5.5 Map of chromium content in drinking water in Southern Ontario demonstrating highly variable concentrations. (From *BMJ Open*. 2017;7(5):e014821. doi: https://doi.org/10.1136/bmjo-pen-2016-014821)

we've fired several bullets, have addressed all the reviewers' concerns, and have reapplied. We are hopeful that we will soon get at least one set of hair samples of every patient for a cross-sectional study, the cannonball awaiting to be fired. The beauty of the CKiD study is that it will allow us to assess for all covariates that have been measured. The process of firing bullets before cannonballs may be longer than just one cannonball, but it is essential for you to assess the likelihood of success before spending all of your resources.

If I had initially followed "fire bullets then cannonballs," I could have avoided this embarrassing review. It's a perfect example of why presenting a big idea without the appropriate foundation is sometimes not a good idea.

How do you ensure you avoid this mistake?

Start with a thorough literature search. Perhaps even consider writing an unsolicited in-depth review of a topic that you want to study. One sneaky way I do this, which is highly educational for an undergraduate or graduate student, is to ask the learner to establish a database using EndNote X8 (this is the reference software that I use). You can store the PDFs of the manuscripts in the database. Typically, I ask that the learner summarizes the main findings in a Word document, and then we meet to give all the available literature some structure. In an attempt to organize the existing summaries in a manner which is structured by themes, topics, and individual chapters, this provides you with an excellent template for writing a review. Your structuring of the database already provides you with a structure for the review. The initial effort of organizing your data will increase your efficiency and assist in easily firing your bullet. This may seem like a small piece of advice, but you will note that writing a review from such a database is a total joy and can be done in only a few hours, as all the information is already structured at your fingertips!

For your grant application, do check that you have ample pilot studies available to support your central hypothesis. These don't necessarily have to be completed all by yourself. You do want to have an impressive amount of supporting documents to avoid that the reviewers accuse you of a fishing expedition (meaning that you have a wild idea without pilot information that renders your hypothesis more likely to be successful). Moreover, you have to demonstrate that the issue matters. For instance, let us look at some valid facts regarding CKD and related matters. It is no secret that there is a lot of oxidative stress in CKD and many individuals are aware that zinc and selenium supplements are widely available; however, at the same time, there is just no information demonstrating whether or not supplementation may provide better outcomes. Correspondingly, Dr. Tonelli's group has done a prospective study in adult dialysis patients and shown that selenium and zinc deficiency are associated with earlier death on dialysis. So, identifying and ameliorating this problem may substantially improve the very, very high risk of cardiovascular death of a child or adolescent with end-stage kidney disease. This is extremely helpful for conveying the point that selenium and zinc deficiency matters. Being oblivious to those deficiencies could contribute to the poor prognosis. Given that the biology of zinc and selenium wasting in end-stage kidney disease should be similar in children as with adults, this topic becomes even more important because the cardiovascular risk of an 18-year-old is about as high as that of an 80-year-old without CKD.

It is hoped that the behavior of accumulating data from small, expendable projects is vitally important as a foundation for a large project. It is typical that an ambitious, young researcher wants to solve a huge problem. However, such ideas, no matter how brilliant they are, rarely flourish and get funded without the necessary legwork. So, if you have a great idea, gather all available literature and design small pilot projects to prove your concept. Publish the proof of concept. Then, perform more pilot studies, publish them, consider a review as well, until you have a solid foundation to make a logical, simple, and straightforward grant for your main idea. *Fire bullets* and, only thereafter, *the cannonball*.

Chapter 6
Productive Paranoia

Productively paranoid leaders do:

1. "They *build (cash) reserves* and buffers to prepare for unexpected events and bad luck *before* they happen.
2. They *bound three kinds of risk – Death Line risk, Asymmetric risk, and Uncontrollable risk.*
3. *They zoom out, then zoom in,* remaining hyper vigilant to sense changing conditions and respond effectively" [1].

Here is a multiple-choice question: If you were to go on a 20-day trip to the Himalayas, which oxygen supply would you bring?

(a) 20 days
(b) 30 days
(c) 40 days
(d) 60 days

I think it goes without saying that nobody would bring only 20-days' worth of oxygen for a 20-day trip. Obviously, the altitude of the Himalayas requires oxygen. You may encounter unexpected delays or problems and not having any extra oxygen would imply a death sentence. Depending on your risk behavior and safety needs, you may bring twice or thrice the amount needed. Roald Amundsen brought 3 tons of supplies for his Antarctica excursion, whereas Scott brought only 1 ton of supplies. Consequently, Amundsen had

© Springer Nature Switzerland AG 2019
G. Filler, R. Nagra, *Becoming a Successful Scholar*,
https://doi.org/10.1007/978-3-030-24448-4_6

plenty of reserves and made it back safely, while Scott's entire team perished.

In your career, you have to do the exact same and exercise precaution or *productive paranoia*. For instance, if you become an assistant professor at the University of Western Ontario, you have to publish approximately ten papers in the 7 years to your promotion to associate professor. How many papers would you budget per year? Of course, at least two! If you do not meet the requirements for promotion, the hospital and the university bylaws result in your termination. You have to be promoted within the timeline to maintain your good standing. If you budget for one paper and then have a pregnancy and maternity leave, you can get a 3-year extension. However, it is well described that there will be some downtime before and after the maternity leave, and you will still end up behind your target. Other unexpected issues may arise that further curtail your productivity. Personally, I would budget for three papers a year to be well within the deadline, but I do also acknowledge that this is a personal preference. I believe it may also be good advice to have at least two papers a year, still allowing for you to be ahead of schedule and to easily be able to account for any bumps down the road.

Build reserves by collecting low-hanging fruit. A case report is not that bad! You can learn a lot from case reports. The clinical case report has a long-standing tradition in the medical literature. While its scientific significance is diminishing, as more advanced research methods evolve, cases reports remain popular in many medical journals.

Why is that? Several case reports may enable a recognizable pattern that leads to the description of a new disease. If you work in an academic institution as a pediatrician, you will likely find at least one new diagnosis in your lifetime. For example, Willem Proesmans described a case of a toddler with Down's syndrome who presented with severe hypercalcemia, hypercalciuria, and medullary nephrocalcinosis [2]. Several other case reports followed. Seven years later, this association was recognized as a disease entity and became known as the Proesmans syndrome [3].

It is undeniable that there are limitations to case reports, as they may not be generalizable. Other limitations include the danger of over-interpretation, publication bias, the retrospective nature of the case report, and distraction of the readers when focusing on the unusual. However, when considering instances where other research designs are not possible to generate, case reports provide valuable in-depth understanding and have immense educational value. Often, the case of a single patient allows researchers and scientists to make observations that are missed in clinical trials, especially in rare diseases. Although randomized trials are now considered the gold standard in medicine-based research, the value of case reports is indispensable, as they generate new hypotheses and stimulate further research. The future prospects of the case report could possibly be in new applications of the genre, for instance, case report databases available online and open access for clinicians and researchers.

The other significant trend in research is individualized medicine or *precision medicine*. It has been proposed that the N-of-1 clinical trial is the ultimate strategy for individualizing medicine. N-of-1 or single subject clinical trials consider an individual patient as the sole unit of observation in a study investigating the efficacy or side-effect profiles of different interventions. I published such a case when witnessing a profound and reversible effect of testosterone in a patient with CKD and hypergonadotropic hypogonadism on renal function. The result was causative because it could be repeated with repeated exposure. We performed extensive studies using novel methods to measure renal blood flow and found an impact of testosterone on renal blood flow. This then resulted in the resurfacing of an old discovery that testosterone receptors are expressed on the kidney's afferent arteriole [4]. This stimulated new research on the impact of testosterone on renal function, which is important as while CKD is more prevalent in females, the incidence of end-stage kidney disease is much higher in males. It may even explain some of the differences in life expectancy between men and women. The ultimate goal of an N-of-1 trial is to determine the optimal or best intervention for an individual patient using objective data-driven criteria. Such trials can leverage study designs and statistical techniques associated with standard population-based clinical trials, including randomization, washout and crossover periods, as well as placebo controls. Despite their obvious appeal and extensive use in educational settings, N-of-1 trials have been used sparingly in medical and general clinical settings. It could be argued that N-of-1 trials demand serious attention among health research and clinical care communities given the contemporary focus on *precision medicine*.

While many established journals ban case reports as they are rarely cited and may diminish the impact factor of the journal, specific journals have emerged that are purposefully designed for case reports. One such example of a high-impact journal is *BMJ Case Reports*, which only requires a subscription to publish.

Another reason for the need for stringent use of available resources is the competitiveness of grant funding for your research projects. It requires funds to conduct the necessary studies. If you fall behind with grant funding, your research progress will ultimately be grounded to a halt. You have to consider that obtaining grant funding nowadays is challenging. Only approximately 11% of applications get funded by large national research institutes.

Bind Three Risks

Successful scholars should be exceedingly cautious regarding how they approach and manage risk, although there is a tendency to not pay a lot of attention to the risks involved. In particular, there are three categories of risk that they give consideration to:

1. *Death line risk:* Jim Collins and Morten T. Hansen define the "death line" using their metaphor of the Himalaya trip: it is the altitude above which the oxygen concentration is too low to support human life. How does this apply to being a scholar? Scholars should use productive para-

noia to manage their time and energy effectively, so they are always above this line. Let us illustrate this with some examples.

Imagine you have a position as an assistant professor in a university that requires your promotion to associate professor within a given time frame (usually 5–7 years). You know at the beginning of your appointment through the university documents what will be required for promotion. Let us say, you should have seven to ten publications as first or senior author in international peer-reviewed journals. Let us also assume that the university will not grant you an extension unless there are some extenuating circumstances. At Schulich School of Medicine and Dentistry at the University of Western Ontario, you can get a one-time extension of 3 years for maternity leave or major illness. Would you budget one publication per year? Hardly! You would be operating above the death line with no oxygen! There will always be unforeseen situations. Your father may fall gravely ill, and you may need to take time off for his care. Your health or family circumstances may require you to reduce your productivity. Do you want to end up with four papers after 5 years, and then suddenly be faced with the need for another three to six in just 1 year, because everything has to be submitted 1 year prior to the deadline? Probably not! Budgeting two to three papers per annum is definitely a good idea.

Another example: You carry multiple small grants for your research and decide to hire a research assistant. To get somebody good, you have to offer them a lengthy contract. Do you start to hire when you have your first $10,000 which may only last you a few months? When do you reapply for more funding? It may be necessary to employ somebody without having the funding for the entire duration of the planned working relationship, but you need to have a suitable buffer for the *likely* event that your grant funding application will not be accepted. It is also important to consider the need for severance payments, especially if the employee is subject to union rules and already has a long history of employment with the institution. Make a budget with a wide margin in order to be able to operate above your death line and prepare for unexpected costs, just like you would be equipped with enough oxygen on your expedition to Mount Everest.

Being constructively paranoid allows you to stay away from unforeseen risks. Be aware that unexpected events may cause a severely damaged reputation. Success does not come from risk; it comes from being prepared and knowing your capabilities and strengths. This hazardous line of either having breathable "oxygen" available or not is a risk you must always remain far from – if you travel at the death line, you risk losing it all.

2. *Asymmetric risks:* These risks are the ones where the downside and possible consequences of a project or task diminish any possible positive outcomes. It is easy to get distracted by the possible prospects of a risk; however, you must be careful to analyze all possible outcomes. If fate is on your side, the gamble you take might have a small chance of working out, but is it worth a much more significant risk? Successful scholars do not jeopardize their professional reputation for a little benefit but, instead, are always aware of all the risks involved. To be successful, you must be mindful of what goals you wish to accomplish and plan ahead of time accordingly, so you are not forced to take risks that could be detrimental to your career.

Let us consider an example: An international society wants you to assemble a group of international experts to write a practice guideline in the society's journal. The community has a clear strategic plan that calls for two to three practice guidelines per year. There are strict rules about equal distribution of contributors based on expertise and geographical location. You know from the society's publication committee that the society is behind schedule. The particular topic requires that you find new collaborators with whom you have never worked before. I have written practice guidelines; they require an incredible amount of work. To complete these practice guidelines with a couple well-known collaborators with whom there was a solid history of mutual publications took 1½ year [5]. So would you accept such a task? The answer should be no. As a successful scholar, you must be able to weigh the good and bad outcomes against each other and use your judgment to decipher whether the risk would be worth the reward. You already established that with a known team of co-authors with a strong past history the task could not be accomplished on time, let alone attempting to do the same task with new collaborators. The pros and cons of taking on this task with an unknown new team are asymmetrical and cannot be calculated. Either ask for a reasonable time frame and put in some checks and balances (such as the society's commitment to hosting regular meetings of the new team and the ability to withdraw) or simply walk away from a deal that is not "win-win."

3. *Uncontrollable risk:* This is a risk which cannot be restrained and where the outcome may be unmanageable. Obviously, this is never the preferred path. Exceptional cases may be heard about where an uncontrolled risk was taken, and a positive outcome may be achieved, but for the majority of cases, this may lead to catastrophe. Do not get fooled by the single story of success of an individual who took an uncontrollable risk. If you look at the majority of successful individuals and enterprises, the key to their triumph is not the one considerable risk they took, but rather the carefully calculated steps they took to achieve small goals one at a time are the cipher to their triumph. If you cannot control the consequences of your actions, you are putting your scholarly success in the hands of chance, an ineffective strategy and an unmerited gamble.

Consider a stool. For milking, farmers used to use a one-legged stool. Imagine, that one leg brakes. You would land in the dirt (Fig. 6.1).

Many mentors teach you to focus on your academic career, to become the world expert about a small, well-defined,

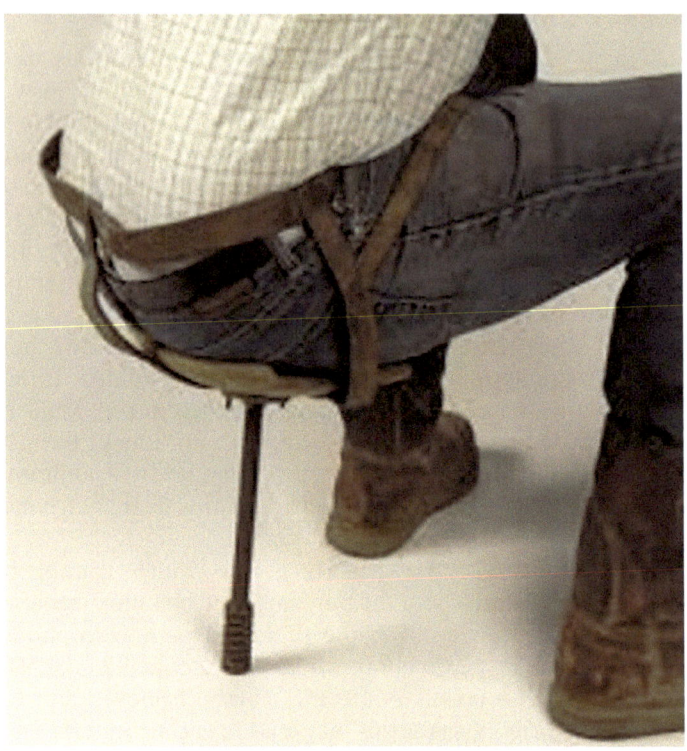

FIGURE 6.1 One-legged stool used for milking cows

highly specialized question. I have never embraced that advice. If the proposed research field question did not work out, the risk of putting all your eggs in one basket would simply be too substantial.

It is almost the norm that you need to modify your topic during the research process. You can never be sure of what you may find. You may find too much data and need to narrow your focus or too little and need to broaden your focus. This is a normal part of the research process. When researching, you may not wish to change your topic, but you may decide that some other aspect of the topic is more interesting or manageable.

Let us say you want to become the world expert on a new biomarker for measuring renal function. You may have multiple candidates, but one really stands out, and then you focus all of your efforts on that one biomarker. After writing numerous grants, bringing various studies through ethics, and publishing a number of papers, it turns out that the biomarker of your choice is strongly affected by inflammation and should not be used, especially as CKD is an inflammatory disease. Now what? It obviously becomes futile to continue to work on this biomarker, yet you have to complete your work for your grants, with no hope for additional publications.

The likelihood for publishing a negative result is remote. In 1990, 30% of papers were published with negative results; however, today, only 14% of papers are published in which you failed to prove your hypothesis [6]. I personally regret this, as negative results are very important. We strive to find the truth: we do not strive to publish papers. Ideally, research protocols are all registered in international repositories like trials.gov, and the results are made public so that the world can build on the cumulative knowledge and other researchers do not repeat the mistakes that were already made.

I always design my studies so that they can have a multitude of possible questions and angles for analysis. Nonetheless, I stick to the protocol, and more and more often, I register and publish the trial designs. However, you always want to have some additional options so that you can deliver. If something goes wrong and you have only one leg to stand on, this is hardly where you want to be (Fig. 6.2).

As the age-old saying goes, never put all your eggs in one basket.

Zoom Out, Zoom In

You will inevitably run into problems. You are not alone if you get completely stuck on a project and feel defeated. But then what?

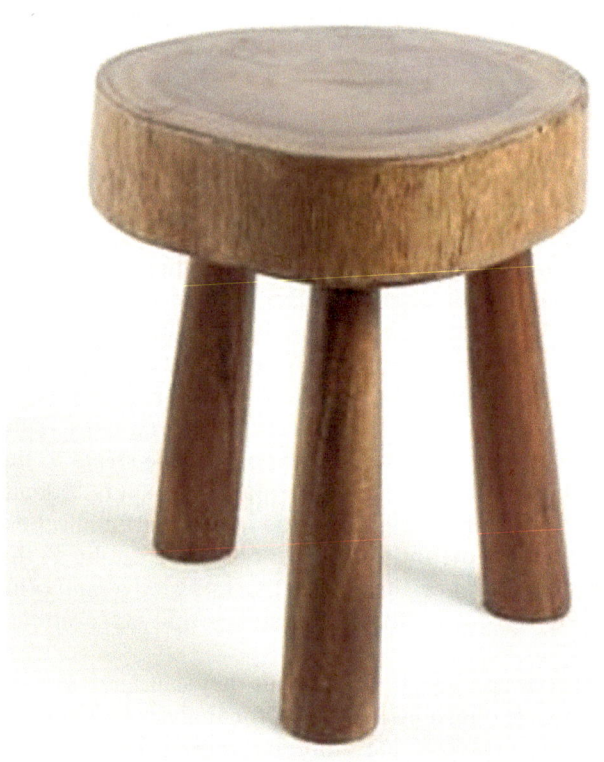

FIGURE 6.2 If you have three different legs on your stool, one can break away, but you won't land in the manure

To answer this question, let us go back to Amundsen. We used Jim Collin's example of the race to the South Pole. However, Roald Amundsen initially did not plan to go to the South Pole. His goal was to conquer the *North* Pole. Unfortunately, with his pedantic and careful planning, he was too late for that excursion. The first group to reach the Geographic North Pole is either Frederick Cook and his two Inuit men, Aapilak and Ittukusuk, or Robert Edwin Peary, Matthew Henson, and four Inuit women: Ootah, Seegloo, Egingway, and Ooqueah. We believe that Amundsen knew about Fredrick Cook's excursion. He did not want to waste careful planning and have all his efforts be in vain, so he *zoomed out*, and decided to conquer the South Pole instead. However, all of the knowledge he obtained from his careful studies about equipment, the 17-mile march, and how not to cross the line of exhaustion were all still applicable for his new goal. As we have learned earlier, he succeeded, and his team returned home without a frozen toe.

When Amundsen was faced with the possibility of a dead end and a floundering goal, he *zoomed out*. Similarly, in your scholarly career, you need to be able to change the lens you use to view your situation. The perspective you embrace when dealing with unexpected barriers can either hinder or benefit the following decisions you make. It is easy to become too focused on the minuscule details of a project, but this can severely hamper your ability to strategically assess possible pathways to your goals. If you are too *zoomed in*, especially when dealing with unexpected situations, it is easy to become frustrated and overlook solutions that are obvious if you simply *zoom out*. Successful scholars can use a wider-angle lens to assess how they should be reacting in certain situations. By *zooming out*, you are able to remain self-aware of changing circumstances, allowing you to be prepared to tackle unexpected problems.

Before I talk more about the concept of *zooming out*, let me provide you with a little background based on my personal experience. In Germany where I trained, you are required to write a medical thesis in addition to your degree as a medical doctor in order to work in an academic health sciences center. Very early in medical school, I was introduced to the outstanding team of transplant surgeons in Hannover, Germany. I was accepted into Rudolph Pichlmayr's group and learned how to perform a bone marrow transplant in the rat and how to perform both donor and recipient surgeries for an auxiliary heart transplant and a pancreas transplant. I transplanted 400 rats to become bone marrow-chimeric animals, and I transplanted 200 hearts and 200 pancreases. The idea was that by exchanging the dendritic cells of the donor with those of the recipient, the organ rejection would be ameliorated. We used congenic rat strains for those experiments. Unfortunately, the method was only able to avoid rejection if there was only a class II histoincompatibility. Fortunately, I got the required three papers from those experiments, wrote my thesis, and successfully defended it. I finished just in time before my growing rat allergy rendered me incapable of performing any additional rat surgeries. Today, an EPI pen is needed if I encounter the saliva of rats.

Fortunately, I got into my residency program, and I forgot all about research. At first, I was accepted into an abdominal and transplant surgery program. In Germany, there is not a big difference in the remuneration of different physician specialties. As a consequence, pediatrics was the most sought-after specialty. Being a boomer, born in one of the highest birth-rate years, the training programs could pick the residents from the top 1% of medical school graduates for pediatrics. Unfortunately, I did not make it. After only a few days, the program in Hannover sought a locum pediatrics resident for 1 year. I took it. It was what I wanted to do. Fortunately, they kept me beyond that 1 year.

At that time, the program in Hannover performed all the liver transplants in children for Germany and Turkey. We performed about 50 liver transplants a year and another 25 kidney transplants annually. I got onto the transplant ward because of my past training. As a resident, you were on-call 3 days of the week. You were not allowed to go home until 7 PM the next day. I was the only resident on the transplant ward. Tacrolimus was not invented yet. We used cyclosporine, and many children developed vanishing bile duct syndrome. Rejection episodes were not uncommon. You can imagine, it was busy. After 1 year on that ward before my next rotation was about to begin, my professor (Professor Johannes Brodehl) cited me into his office for a performance review. I did not write a single case report in that year. All my research was at a standstill. You can imagine how my heart was racing when I entered his office, especially as my ongoing residency was dependent on the performance review.

He said, "You established yourself as an excellent clinician. You lead the ward rounds excellently. You are a great teacher to undergraduate students. However, you suck with your research performance. We will keep you, but smarten up, or you will be out of here. There are many who would gladly take your spot." Do not worry, we later became friends, and I owe him a great deal. However, at the time, I was devastated.

Here is the situation:

- Continuing transplant research in the rat model was hazardous to my life due to my allergies.
- The transplant research was immunological and basic, and I simply would not have enough time doing residency for this, even without my rat allergy.
- It became quite clear during that 1 year that I was drawn to nephrology. I enjoyed going down to the dialysis unit regularly, and I just loved the pathophysiology of the kidney. I wanted to become a pediatric nephrologist, so obviously I should be doing research in pediatric nephrology.
- I had to come up with a plan on how to do research that was compatible with the busy life of a resident in the 1980s.

I definitely had to *zoom out.* One of the diseases that I still do not understand was childhood nephrotic syndrome. I should add that at that time the center in Hannover, a total of eight randomized controlled trials were performed on childhood nephrotic syndrome, and at the time, I was heavily involved in recruiting patients. So, I thought, this is it! This is what I could do research in!

What did I do? I booked another appointment with Professor Brodehl. This time, I was leading the conversation. I knew that he was very interested in nephrotic syndrome. I stroked his ego by asking him to point me to the world's leading researcher in childhood nephrotic syndrome. As he was doing research in childhood nephrotic syndrome using an epidemiological and randomized controlled clinical trials approach, I knew he would need someone to research the underlying pathophysiology of the condition. I told him that I wanted to do this and asked him whom I should spend time with. I offered to apply for a postdoc and go abroad, provided that he would keep the spot in the training program for me and would consider hiring me later to develop this research branch in his department. He ended up pointing me to perhaps the most influential person in my life, Professor Martin Barratt at Great Ormond Hospital in London, England. Not only did he make the introductions, but he actually helped me write the post-doc application to the German government. Luckily, I was funded even though I did not have any research in this field. I was awarded a 2-year salaried post-doc and off I went.

I have to say that this move was the best thing that could happen to me. Professor Barratt was Dean of Medicine at that time. Nonetheless, he greeted me on arrival personally. He said, "I am Martin." He was a person of medium-tall structure, impeccable posture, impeccable clothing, coming across as a person you must bow for in respect for his intimidating status. When I met and told him, "It is my deepest honor to meet you, Professor Barratt", he shook his index finger and said, "That is Martin." I replied, "Professor Barratt, I could *never address* you by your first name." He replied, "Everyone does!", and indeed everyone did, although from the respect in their voice, they may as well have been addressing the Pope! This gesture of kindness was incredible. It lowered all my defenses towards any criticism that he had about my performance.

When you may feel defeated, ensure you have taken the time to assess your position and take care to be critical of what you may need to change and what you have the ability to change in your project: *zoom out*. When there is total clarity about your purpose and goals, only then should you *zoom in* and bring the details of your project into sharp focus. *Zooming in* allows you to focus on the specifics of your projects and perfect the details. However, it is important to remain vigilant of the fact that you may need to *zoom out* at any point in time, and this will always remain an important skill. Being productively paranoid and aware of how your situation may be changing allows you to plan ahead and overcome obstacles you encounter, but if you do face challenges, *zooming out* remains important in persevering through them. In other words, if you are stuck, do not toss everything into the garbage, but salvage what works, and *zoom out* on how you may apply your assets. Then *zoom* back *in* once you have determined your goal and purpose. Just like Amundsen, the North Pole fell, but the South Pole was his to reach for.

References

1. https://www.willmancini.com/blog/leading-above-the-death-line.
2. Proesmans W, et al. Hypercalcaemia, hypercalciuria and nephrocalcinosis in Down syndrome. Pediatr Nephrol. 1995;9(1):112–4.
3. Ramage IJ, et al. Hypercalcaemia in association with trisomy 21 (Down's syndrome). J Clin Pathol. 2002;55(7):543–4.
4. Filler G, et al. Is Testosterone Detrimental to Renal Function? Kidney Int Rep. 2016;1(4):306–10.
5. Filler G, Melk A, Marks SD. Practice recommendations for the monitoring of renal function in pediatric non-renal organ transplant recipients. Pediatr Transplant. 2016;20(3):352–63. https://doi.org/10.1111/petr.12685.
6. https://www.economist.com/news/leaders/21588069-scientific-research-has-changed-world-now-it-needs-change-itself-how-science-goes-wrong.

Chapter 7
Return on Luck

Across all the research we've conducted for this book and our previous books regarding what makes companies great (which has involved investigating the histories of 75 major corporations), we've never found a single instance of sustained performance due simply to pure luck. Yet also true, we've never studied a single great company devoid of luck events along its journey. Neither extreme—it's all luck or luck plays no role—has the evidence on its side. A far better fit with the data is a synthesizing concept, return on luck [1].

You may think that some researchers have just gotten very lucky. However, in Collins' and Hansen's book *Great by Choice*, there was no evidence for more luck among the highly successful and resilient companies. Collins and Hansen coined the concept of "return on luck." Their research showed that the great companies were not generally luckier than other comparing companies – they did not get more good luck, less lousy luck, significant spikes of luck, or better timing of luck. Instead, they got a higher return on luck and made more of their luck than others had. Evidently, the critical question is not "Will you get lucky?" but "What will you do with the luck that you get?"

In my career, I had luck several times. I want to give you some examples.

In transplantation, there were a few breakthroughs with the immune-suppressive medications. The achievements of the 60s and 70s were mostly due to the use of azathioprine

© Springer Nature Switzerland AG 2019
G. Filler, R. Nagra, *Becoming a Successful Scholar*,
https://doi.org/10.1007/978-3-030-24448-4_7

and steroids. However, while unusual long-term graft surviv-
als could be achieved with these drugs for up to 35 years
after kidney transplantation, 50% of the grafts were lost in
the first year. The immunosuppression was too weak. When
Borel and Feurer introduced a new drug called cyclosporine,
a calcineurin inhibitor, in 1977, [2] it was a major game-
changer. One-year graft survival increased to 90%.
Unfortunately, the drug had substantial cosmetic side effects,
especially hypertrichosis (excessive hair growth) and gingi-
val hyperplasia (enlargement of the gums). You could tell if
a child was on cyclosporine from 20 yards away. In the late
1980s, Fujisawa found another drug (also a calcineurin inhibitor) which later became known as tacrolimus. Results were
quite favorable in adult transplantation. Unfortunately, the
company insisted on a 2:1 randomization for the trials. This
type of trial introduces a bias that always favors the innova-
tor's drug. In the mid-1990s, the time was prime to start conducting a similar study among children. However, we needed
to conduct a proper scientific study for tacrolimus with a 1:1
randomization and not a 2:1 randomization. Concurringly, I
was extremely lucky to be in charge of what was then the
largest pediatric renal transplant program in Germany.
Fujisawa GmbH, the European branch of Fujisawa Inc., was
based in Japan but also happened to be in Germany. It is
absolutely a lucky coincidence that I met some high-ranking
Fujisawa leaders at a conference. The attitude in Germany
was against tacrolimus because of reports of diabetes and
lymphoproliferative disease in the United States among
adult renal transplant recipients. Owing to the desire to demonstrate a superior ability to control rejection, exposure to
tacrolimus was too high for the initial studies. Moreover, the
headquarters of the company that introduced cyclosporine
was in Basel, Switzerland, and strongly influenced the community of German transplant physicians to favor cyclosporine. At the same time, Fujisawa was determined to conduct
a randomized control trial in children.

Indeed, I was very fortunate to have had the opportunity
to introduce myself to Fujisawa leadership; however, what is

more important was how I used that opportunity to get a *return on my luck*. I was able to convince them that I could assemble an international consortium of pediatric renal transplant centers in Europe, where I made many friends among pediatric nephrology centers due to my training in the United Kingdom. The company also only wanted a 6-month randomized controlled trial. They insisted on a 2:1 randomization.

I went ahead and contacted my friends: Richard Trompeter (London, UK), Nicholas J.A. Webb (Manchester, UK), Alan R. Watson (Nottingham, UK), David V. Milford (Birmingham, UK), Gunnar Tyden (Stockholm, Sweden), Ryszard Grenda (Warsaw, Poland), Jan Janda (Prague, Czech Republic), David Hughes (Glasgow, UK), Jochen H.H. Ehrich (Hannover, Germany), Bernd Klare (Munich, Germany), Graziella Zacchello (Padova, Italy), Inge Bjorn Brekke (Oslo, Norway), Mary McGraw (Bristol, UK), Ferenc Perner (Budapest, Hungary), Lucian Ghio (Milan, Italy), Egon Balzar (Vienna, Austria), Styrbjörn Friman (Gothenburg, Sweden), Rosanna Gusmano (Palermo, Italy), and Jochen Stolpe (Rostock, Germany). We met at international conferences, and I was extremely fortunate to be chosen as the leader of this group, which later became known as the European Paediatric Renal Transplant Study Group. We set our own list of demands and started negotiating with Fujisawa. We clearly demonstrated that we could transplant 200 children, as they requested, within a couple of years. After tough negotiations, we won and got a 1:1 randomization, as well as an open-label, follow-up study for 4 years. And so, the trial went ahead and was completed successfully.

Of course, it is desirable to be the first author when you lead a study. However, I experienced some bad luck. Even as the leader of the European Paediatric Renal Transplant Study Group, I was not the first author from the first paper of this trial. This is because we made rules about authorship at the very beginning. To avoid a center bias, we limited the number of patients that could be enrolled in the trial from each center to 32 (out of the total 200 patients). Berlin, where

I was at the time, had a head start and started recruiting as early as July 1996. Most unfortunately, two children that were randomized to the cyclosporine arm of the study were given the drug from the pharmacy, rather than the study's cyclosporine. Both London and Berlin recruited 32 patients, but these 2 children from our center were disqualified. That is why Richard Trompeter was the first author of the first paper, even though I did most of the writing. I do recommend that you establish the order of authorship ahead of time and adhere to it. Today, in a situation like this, you can have two co-principal authors in some journals.

Despite using a 1:1 randomization, we still found a significant advantage of tacrolimus with lower rejection rates and better graft function at 6 months, 1 year, and 4 years. The 1-year and the 4-year data, I was fortunate enough to write up because I was leading the open-label follow-up study. It would be wrong to say that I completely lived by the principles outlined in this book at that time because I did not get the highest return on luck that I could have if I did. If I lived by the principled outlined in this book, I should have published the results after 2 years *and* 3 years of follow-up in addition to the papers that were published. Moreover, I should have written additional papers using subgroup analyses. The yield of three highly cited papers from this randomized control trial is okay, but indeed not the maximum that could have been achieved. I was lucky, but this goes to show that your return on luck is of ultimate prominence. The challenges of exploiting the unique and powerful data obtained was hampered by the fact that I moved continents because of leadership challenges in Berlin and a unique opportunity in Ottawa, where they were looking for a chief of pediatric nephrology. Also, it was extremely difficult to get the long-term follow-up data from each of the centers. I had to use my personal relationship to maintain the flow of data. As an academic clinician, you rarely get the opportunity for more than one randomized controlled trial in your lifetime. Had I known what I know today, there would have been at least another three papers.

Nonetheless, this study became highly influential. The vast majority of all pediatric renal transplant centers now use tacrolimus as their mainstream calcineurin inhibitor.

Let me give you another example of the more recent past. For some time, I have been collaborating with my friend Doctora Mara Medeiros from Frederico, Gomez Hospital, in Mexico City. She introduced me to one of her fellows at the biannual conference of the *International Pediatric Transplantation Association* IPTA at San Francisco in 2015, Ana Catalina Alvarez Elias. Mara suggested that Ana Catalina should spend a 3-month research fellowship with me. She told me that Ana Catalina is extremely talented and hardworking. Ana Catalina came in the fall and was a real star. In 3 months, we published five papers based on existing study materials that I had ready for analysis. During her stay, we developed a friendship for life. Ana Catalina later introduced me to some of her powerful friends, especially Maria Ferris from Chapel Hill, North Carolina. Maria was kind enough to introduce me to two major studies she was doing. One involved a longitudinal study of transition of pediatric nephrology patients into adult care. The other one is called PICCOLO MONDO, which is an offspring of a worldwide dialysis study of the Renal Research Institute (RRI) in New York. She asked me to help her to analyze complex data that Ana Catalina had been working on that was of almost 400 children receiving hemodialysis around the world. I was able to streamline the message, and we are very close to getting this paper into the *Journal of Pediatrics*, which is the highest-ranking pediatrics journal. I treasure and foster this new friendship and look forward to many more collaborations. Without that friendship to Ana Catalina, who I visited frequently in Mexico (and even met her parents), I would have never been able to get into these large studies that opened incredible treasures for me. Do invest in such academic friendships as this will lead to more academic opportunities. You may also want to consider some investments. For instance, I let Ana Catalina stay at my house for free. This small investment resulted in a huge return and I have Mexican friends for good. I invest in that friendship in multiple ways, including the offering of co-authorship when appropriate opportunities arise. I receive a return on luck by continuing to invest, rather than hoping I am always just "lucky." We are never just handed achievements and greatness by fate: we must take the wheel and steer our own destiny toward a path where we can continue to reap the rewards, rather than hoping for opportunities and lucky chances to come to us.

Let me add one more piece to this story. Ana Catalina was facing incredible competition for a job in Mexico. Ana Catalina also achieved incredible return on luck. She basically told me that despite her additional research training, her outlook for an academic position was grim. Because of the five papers and substantial productivity that originated there after once I had taught her how to do scientific publications, she was awarded the one vacant clinician scientist position at Frederico Gomez Hospital in Mexico City. She is currently undergoing additional training at the University of Toronto, but her path as a highly successful clinician scientist is clearly laid out.

The message is simple: opportunities need to be looked out for and seized. Luck alone does not produce outcomes. Many people get lucky; however, the art lies in the ability to see the opportunities and to make the most out of it. It is the execution of the opportunities that arise from luck that makes all the difference. Be prepared to make a little investment, and the returns will be substantial. We will talk more about weapons of influence when you are working with others later, but the impact of the weapon of influence of reciprocity specifically is extremely powerful, especially in relation to getting your return on luck. Do not stumble when luck arrives; execute superbly and effectively because the opportunity may not arise again.

Let me elaborate on this with another example: I am certain that I was not the only person that Fujisawa Inc. approached when they felt the time had come for expanding the randomized trials comparing cyclosporine and tacrolimus. I was lucky because I was in the right country at the right time, and Berlin then happened to have one of the largest pediatric renal transplant programs. When this opportunity arose, I was able to quickly assemble a plan, call my friends to get their verbal commitment, and promptly and effectively demonstrate (a) sufficient numbers to meet the goal of 100 patients per arm, (b) the willingness to collaborate, and (c) the willingness to invest extra work to make this happen. Do not be shy of this small commitment. Take some time to reflect on the words of no one less than Thomas A. Edison, the inventor of the light bulb which changed the world as we know it forever. He wrote:

> Most people miss opportunities because it is dressed in overalls and looks like work.
>
>   Thomas A. Edison, 1847–1931, famous American inventor and business man.

References

1. https://www.jimcollins.com/concepts/return-on-luck.html.
2. https://www.ncbi.nlm.nih.gov/pubmed/328380.

Chapter 8
The Mindset Helps

My favorite psychologist is Carol S. Dweck, the inventor of the growth mindset. According to her, we basically have two types of people. Those with a fixed mindset and those with a growth mindset. The person with a fixed mindset thinks as follows: "I am either good at this or I am not. When I am frustrated, I give up. I don't like to be challenged. When I fail, I am no good. Tell me, I am smart. If you succeed, I feel threatened. My abilities determine everything." Let us examine this. It is true that you should always build on your strengths. You can only achieve mastery if you develop your talents. Children learn this early in life. Naturally, they invest in their abilities and develop them further in a playful way, whereas when things are challenging, the mind procrastinates and avoids them. The mind is deceiving; it will not motivate you to start a task where it does not actually perceive a 70% likelihood for success. We have talked about this. One strategy to overcome these challenges is to divide the work into small, manageable pieces. The key to overcoming this procrastinating tendency of our minds is by finding our 17-mile marches. However, even when embracing habits that make you more successful, if you have a fixed mindset, it will limit growth. I am unsure though that things are simply black and white, and you have either a growth mindset or a fixed mindset. I am not a psychologist, but I feel as though the extremely absolute way this mindset has been described is not what the

G. Filler, R. Nagra, *Becoming a Successful Scholar*,
https://doi.org/10.1007/978-3-030-24448-4_8

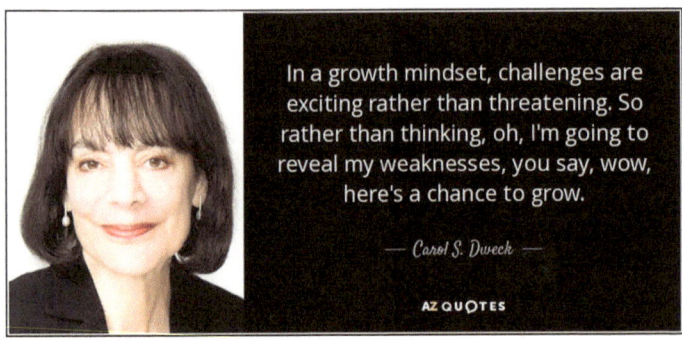

In a growth mindset, challenges are exciting rather than threatening. So rather than thinking, oh, I'm going to reveal my weaknesses, you say, wow, here's a chance to grow.

— *Carol S. Dweck* —

AZ QUOTES

FIGURE 8.1 Carol Dweck's advice on re-framing your thoughts can enable you to face the challenges you face!

average person feels. I feel like most people are stuck somewhere in between the fixed mindset and the growth mindset and do not know how to push themselves closer to the growth mindset.

Carol Dweck propagates the growth mindset, instead of the fixed mindset outlined above. Think as follows: "I can learn anything I want to. When I am frustrated, I persevere. I want to challenge myself. When I fail, I learn. Tell me I try hard. If you succeed, I am inspired. My effort and my attitude determine everything." This is of course not easy. But it is essential. We have to see challenges as opportunities, not as threats. Constantly ask yourself, is this the best I can do? When asking that question, the desire to improve your productivity comes naturally.

I fully confess that developing a growth mindset is not easy, and the examples that I will be listing below are taken from Dr. Dweck's books. But they are very telling, and I recommend embracing them.

- Instead of thinking, "I'm not good at this," try thinking "what am I missing?"
- Instead of giving up, try thinking "I should try a different strategy."
- Instead of stating "It is good enough," ask yourself "is this the best work I can do?"

- Instead of saying "I can't make this any better," consider saying "I can always improve."
- Instead of saying "this is too hard," tell yourself "it will take some time."
- Instead of saying "I made a mistake," tell yourself that "mistakes help me learn."
- Instead of giving up and saying "I just cannot do this," say to yourself "I am going to train my brain."
- Instead of "I will never be that smart," say to yourself "I will learn how to do this."
- If Plan A didn't work, there's always Plan B.
- Instead of telling yourself your friend can do this, tell yourself that you want to learn from them.

Why is this important? If you follow the fixed mindset, you will avoid challenges. You will often see your effort as fruitless and worthless. You will tend to ignore insightful and beneficial negative feedback. The success of others will make you feel threatened, and as a result, you may plateau early on and achieve less than your full potential.

Alternatively, try the following: embrace challenges. Persist in the face of setbacks and obstacles. See effort as a path to mastery, not a mundane and tedious process. Learn from criticism. And find lessons and inspirations in the success of others. The reward is ever higher levels of achievement and a greater sense of free will.

It sounds so easy. It is not. You are threatened in a junior position. You are worried about your own career. You are afraid that you may not get promoted. These perceived threats can paralyze you. As a result, you procrastinate, arrive in Quadrant 3 and 4, and don't seize opportunities.

Let us be frank. You cannot afford that. As we outlined, the boomer babies face fierce competition. I admire the Millennials and Gen-Ys because they have ambition. *You* have Level 5 Ambition. To get bulked down by perceived threats and the success of others is just not an option.

Don't get frustrated. View a rejected paper as an opportunity to make it better. Carefully consider the editors' and reviewers' comments. Address them in a point-to-point fashion in a pedantic approach before resubmitting the paper. Ask yourself two questions to help you focus your editing:

1. So, what?
2. Are the findings generalizable?

Both must have strong answers.

Tell yourself that challenges are opportunities. Question the challenges. Look behind every stone to find opportunities to address your questions in a different manner. Zoom out. The rewards will be sumptuous. There is not sufficient space in this book to really go into a deeper discussion of the psychology of success. However, the mindset is everything.

Chapter 9
Behaviors That Make You More Successful

> Motivation is what gets you started. Habit is what keeps you going.
>
> – Jim Rohn

The habits you keep may be very helpful tools, which are often underestimated, to prevent you from procrastinating and getting on with your work. Your mind plays tricks on you to get you into Quadrant 3 or 4 (urgent but not important or not urgent and not important). In order to start a project or a task, there has to be a perceived likelihood for success of at least 70%. To achieve that, rather than attempting to tackle an entire project at once, start by breaking it down into small chunks, as outlined in "Fanatic Discipline." That is just the start. You can do more to motivate your mind to help you.

For instance, a big task will easily continue to build up and consequently cause you to procrastinate more and more. As the task gets exceedingly more daunting and the larger it is perceived to be, the more you will procrastinate. So why not map it out into many small pieces *as soon as you get it*. Build in buffers as well, so that you can easily get back on track. For instance, you cannot write a whole paper at once, but what you can do is assign yourself 1 week to get all relevant literature.

© Springer Nature Switzerland AG 2019
G. Filler, R. Nagra, *Becoming a Successful Scholar*,
https://doi.org/10.1007/978-3-030-24448-4_9

Using Influencing Tools to Keep You Focused

An individual is more susceptible for interruptions than two or more people

Have you ever procrastinated? The deadline for a task is 4 weeks away, and you do not worry about it that much. It is not a humongous task, but it will require probably north of 8 hours of work. You put it off for 2 weeks, and then you suddenly remember the up-and-coming deadline. The task has grown much prominent. In attempting to avoid confronting this scary project, you procrastinate further, and 1 week later, the task has grown to a mountain. The closer the deadline comes, the more insurmountable the task appears. And then what may happen? You panic 2 days before, pull two all-nighters, and manage to put together a project, but you know the product that you finally submit really is not the best you could have done and definitely does not reflect your potential. Does that sound familiar?

We already talked about determining your 17-mile march, but there is a lot more you can do. We also talked about the psychology of having to have a 70% likelihood chance of success for your mind to initiate an assignment and avoid procrastination. To explain the following section, we need to quickly review these six principles of influence, as defined by Robert Cialdini [1]: *reciprocity, commitment and consistency, social proof, authority, liking, and scarcity.*

- *Reciprocity*: This refers to the urge of a person to return a favor.
- *Commitment and consistency*: If a person commits orally or in writing, to an idea or goal, she or he is more likely to honor that commitment because not completing this goal would be incongruent with their self-image. Even if the original incentive or motivation is removed after the person has already agreed, she or he will continue to honor the commitment.
- *Social proof*: People will copy the behaviors of other people. In Cialdini's book, he cites the famous experiment

where one or more confederates would look up into the sky and bystanders would copy that behavior to see what individuals were trying to see. This can be extrapolated to scholarly work.

- *Authority*: Most unfortunately, this is the most widely used principle of influence. It is also one of the weakest.
- *Liking*: People are easily persuaded by other people that they like. Cialdini cites the marketing of Tupperware in what might now be called viral marketing.
- *Scarcity*: The rarer an item or a behavior, the more individuals will demand it. In Cialdini's book, he refers to the "limited time only" example.

The power of these six principles varies greatly. It is my opinion that commitment and consistency is by far the most powerful, followed by reciprocity. By contrast, it is also of my opinion that authority does not work at all. Let us illustrate these points with examples, and let us talk about how we can use these principles of influence to help us get on with our work.

Firstly, let me clear up why authority is the weakest weapon of influence and should be steered clear of. When I became department chair, I was asked to implement a pay-per-performance system to boost the academic productivity of the department. It was a mundane task to get everyone to agree on principles. We developed over 2 years a detailed performance measurement tool in all domains, clinical, research, teaching, and healthcare leadership and administration. Finally, everyone agreed on it. We then implemented this tool and put approximately 15% of the remuneration at risk. The outcome was devastating. Rather than improving the academic performance, it went down! You cannot expect an improvement in academic performance just for money. There has to be a higher purpose. However, putting a salary at risk is a common tool for the use of *authority* to influence people.

As can be seen from the picture of the paper which was published in *Academic Medicine*, although there was a robust tool implemented for the measurement of performance, performance-based remuneration had *no* effect on the physicians' performances (Fig. 9.1).

Research Report

**Measuring Physicians' Productivity:
A Three-Year Study to Evaluate a New
Remuneration System**

Guido Filler, MD, PhD, Vanessa Burkoski, RN, MScN, DHA, and Gary Tithecott, MD

Abstract

Purpose
To evaluate a new assessment tool measuring physicians' academic productivity and its use in a performance-based remuneration system.

Method
The authors developed an assessment tool based on existing tools to measure productivity. Yearly, from 2008 to 2011, physicians at the University of Western Ontario received a score of up to three points for each of four components (impact, application, scholarly activity, mentorship) in each of four domains (clinical practice, education, research, administration). Scores were weighted by the percentage of time physicians spent on tasks in each domain. Year 1 scores were a baseline. In Years 2 and 3, scores were tied to remuneration. The authors compared scores and associations, accounting for age and academic rank, across the three years.

Results
The 37 participating physicians included 11 assistant, 23 associate, and 4 full professors. The mean weighted total baseline score across all four domains was 7.44. Years 2 and 3 scores were highly correlated with Year 1 scores ($r = 0.85$, Years 1 and 2; $r = 0.89$, Years 1 and 3). Year 2 mean weighted scores did not differ significantly from Year 1 scores. Assistant professors' scores improved significantly between Years 1 and 2 (+1.08, $P < .001$). Lower Year 1 scores were correlated with a greater improvement in scores between Years 1 and 2, and age was negatively correlated with score changes between Years 2 and 3.

Conclusions
Although the tool may be a robust measurement of physicians' productivity, performance-based remuneration had no effect on physicians' overall performance.

FIGURE 9.1 A study evaluating the effectiveness of remuneration to increase performance demonstrates that this method simply does not work

By contrast, *reciprocity* works really well. By working with your colleagues and assisting them in achieving success, you will almost inevitably be rewarded, as there is evidently an underlying obligation to repay your hard work. The functionality of reciprocity is a cross-cultural phenomenon that is a natural part of human nature, as it was evolutionarily beneficial for our ancestors. We also have an obligation to receive, and sometimes what we receive is greater than what we wish or asked for, and this in return cycles back to an even greater desire and urge to repay. As an example, I had the distinct pleasure to co-supervise the PhD of Dr. Shih-Han Susan Huang. She is now an adult nephrologist, MD/ PhD, working as a clinician researcher in our institution. We published multiple papers together during her PhD. From this came a great friendship, and we now discuss multiple research projects and continue to publish together (Fig. 9.2). Each collaboration stimulates new collaboration for the next project. The rule of reciprocity results in ever-increasing mutual productivity. Here is a great tool for how you can simply double your research output.

Another example of *reciprocity* originates from my friendship with Dr. Maria Ferris from the University of North

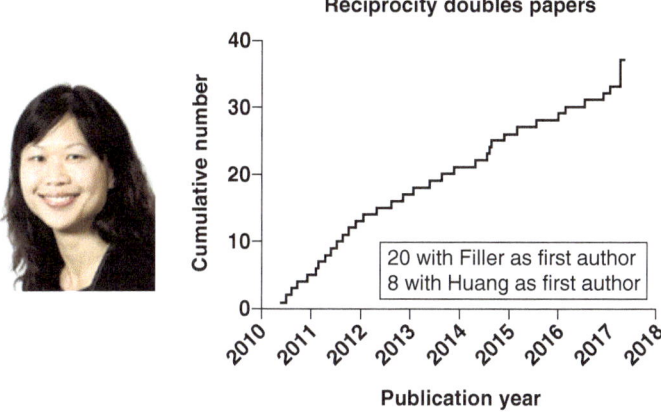

Reciprocity doubles papers

20 with Filler as first author
8 with Huang as first author

FIGURE 9.2 The cumulative amount of papers published since the time Dr. Shih-Han and I began collaborating has more than tripled in less than 10 years

Carolina at Chapel Hill. We involve each other in mutual projects, which gives her and myself access to new research fields and data. The resulting publications emerge much stronger than what could have been accomplished by both highly accomplished individuals alone. Ideally, you want to build a network of collaborations for a worldwide network which will result in convergence of approach to research questions and, ultimately, much higher caliber publications. Good examples of this convergence are the consensus statements on pharmacokinetic monitoring of mycophenolic acid and the practice recommendations in the field of pediatric transplantation. *Reciprocity* is probably the second most powerful principle to grow your research. The current research collaborations are depicted in the Fig. 9.3 below:

Collaborations also help to grow the academic profile of divisions or even departments or even across departments. Unfortunately, I never published the following, but I conducted a simple experiment on collaborations within a single department. I found an online program that would automatically adjust the proximity of different items in relation to the number of connections present between them. I generated a map of the department members based on the publication

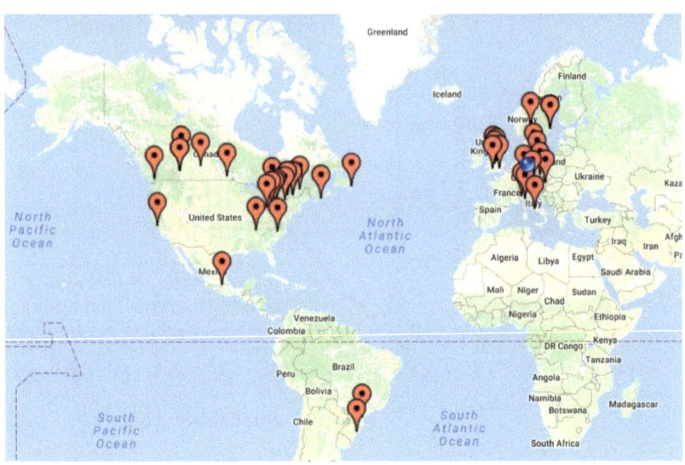

FIGURE 9.3 Locations of current research collaborations

records over 3 years. For each mutual paper, I drew a line. The program automatically pulled collaborators together. I then made the size of the square for each author proportional to the number of publications of the time period. The result was fascinating. There was a direct proportionality between the academic output and the research collaborations. Looking at the Fig. 9.4 below, it is intriguing and amusing that you can almost spot some "organs." To the top is the head, with a neurometabolic and neurogenetic focus. Then there is a heart, focusing on cardiology and intensive care. There is also clearly one kidney. This was all coincidentally the result of the program and had nothing of my doing, but it definitely highlights the notion that collaborations connect academia into one united body.

The principle of *commitment and consistency,* however, is by far the most effective tool. This is actually how we wrote this book. Ravneet and I agreed on the principle and committed ourselves to it. We booked many short 1–2-hour appointments to fit our 17-mile march. We agreed after each meeting to complete manageable individual assignments before the next meeting. Neither of us wanted to disappoint the other,

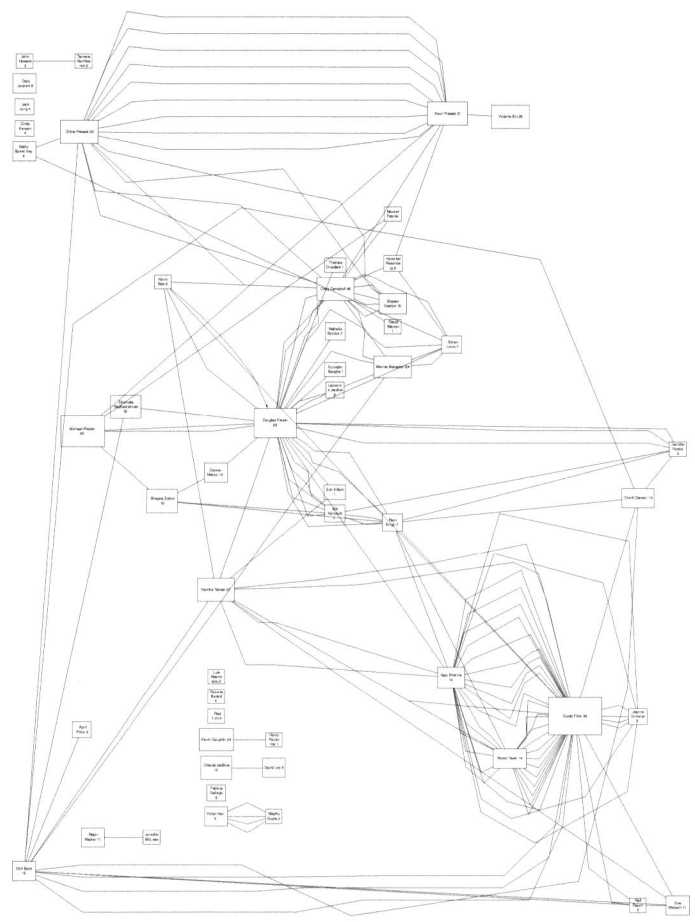

FIGURE 9.4 Research relationships over a 3-year study period (2010–2013) within the Department of Paediatrics at the University of Western Ontario

and we always completed our tasks in full. The psychological impact of not wanting to disappoint your peers is a powerful tool to overcome your own inertia and procrastination.

Use these principles of influence to propel your own research forward:

- When working in a team, you do not want to disappoint or be disappointed. Use *commitment and consistency* to complete more work in a timely fashion.
- Peer pressure can be positive and motivating – your desire not to disappoint others forms the strongest pull to make you provide your deliverables.
- You do not want to disappoint peers. Use this internal motivation as a strong tool to overcome your own procrastination.
- Book appointments with your collaborators at the appropriate 17-mile march intervals. Assign tasks at the end of each session, and quickly review them when you meet again. Never rebuke your peers if they have not completed the assignments. Just say: "Do this by Y rather than by X." There is no need to criticize. At your next meeting, the embarrassment of disappointing you and others depending on their work will likely result in all the tasks being complete.
- Use appropriate software to keep track of your responsibilities. I use MeisterTask, which is a free program, and all your collaborators can download it for free. It even works on tabloids and phones. You assign tasks schedules and deadlines, and it wonderfully keeps your work moving forward. There are many other similar tools, and most of them are free.

The Fight Against the Email Inbox

Time management and an unorganized email inbox are incompatible. Regardless of how many emails you may receive daily, there are essentially only several categories of emails. There are emails which are trash, ideally emails which you should never see. Others that can be categorized as a Quadrant 4 activity are trivia, and you should block them. On the other hand, there are emails which need addressing and require your attention. Ideally, you should organize your emails according to subheadings based on your personal needs, such as entitling them @task, @appointments, and @ InformationForFiling. This allows you to quickly attend to emails that are relevant and actually require a response or some form of action. By adding the "@" sign to the folder names, these subfolders will be organized at the top of the list, thus assisting with quicker access. Beneficially, many software applications are now available that seamlessly should sort through your emails (however, until more rigorous programs are developed, you may unfortunately still find yourself at times having to sort through subheadings to sort out junk).

Making Schedules

Writing a paper requires a lot of steps. You have an idea. You write it down. You then discuss your idea with peers and revise it, making it clearer and more precise. You prepare an ethics submission and prepare a grant application, if applicable. Then you have to address the comments, edits, or changes. You get rejected and resubmit. Then you finally get it approved. You go through the steps of setting up what is needed; for instance, you may need to set up a REDCap® database. While provided free of charge for the members of my institution, there are a lot of necessary steps that must be taken first to get that approved. Then you finally start to collect data. Let us say you are completing a retrospective chart review. If you prospectively enroll patients, it takes a lot of time. After all this, you will finally have the data and be able to start the analysis. You may have to involve a statistician. After this, you finally have results, but the null hypothesis has to be rejected. This might require you to zoom out, reanalyze the data, and rewrite your paper. Find another teachable moment. You get writer's block. You procrastinate, and before you know it, the project is 3 years old and now difficult to publish because the data is old. Research takes a long time. It may even be that someone ends up already publishing your idea. You might as well give up.

Unfortunately, this happens all too often. Only a part of the work that was done gets presented as a poster or platform presentation with a published abstract, and of those, only about ¼ get published [2]. This is sad because there is substantial publication bias. Journals tend to publish positive results but ignore mostly confirmatory papers and are very hesitant to publish negative results. However, it is ever so important to publish the negative results [3]. Mlinarić et al. conclude "Underreporting of negative results introduces bias into the meta-analysis, which consequently misinforms researchers, doctors and policymakers. More resources are potentially wasted on already disputed research that remains unpublished and therefore unavailable to the scientific community. Ethical obligations need to be considered when reporting the results of studies on human subjects as people have exposed themselves to risk with the assurance that the study is performed to benefit others. Some studies disprove the common conception that journal editors preferably publish positive findings, which are considered as more citable. Therefore, all stakeholders, but especially researchers, need to be conscious of disseminating negative and positive findings alike." We could not agree more with this.

However, apart from these ethical considerations, there is an important point to make: You want to publish close to 100% of the studies you undertook. You also want to publish way more than just one or two papers over 2 years. This is why I propose you make schedules: Detailed schedules that are designed to be in different stages of project completion at all times so that you have data ready to analyze every month and, eventually, a paper to submit every month. I believe that this is the only way, other than through collaboration, to have a strong steady (17-mile-march-like) research output. You will remain in Quadrant 2 when you make your schedule.

You can simply use Excel to make your schedules. I use that for the big overview. For more detailed lists, I use MeisterTask (please see below). I am currently working on 17 projects, all of which are in different stages. Some are just at

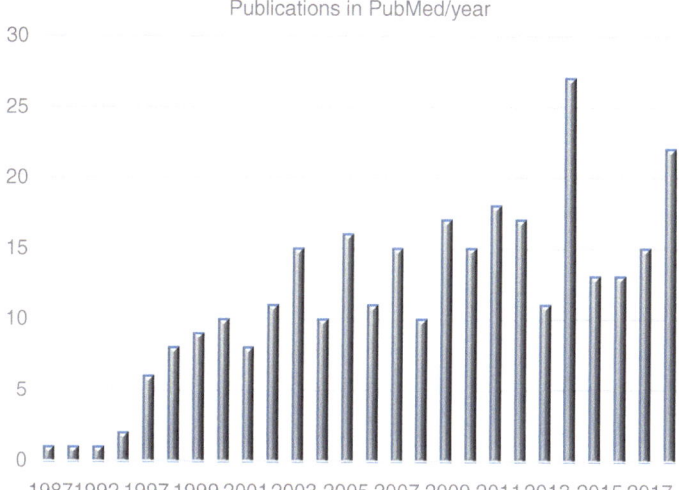

Publications in PubMed/year

FIGURE 9.5 PubMed listed publications of the author. Since 2003, there was an average of 15/year. I have been using the strategies mentioned above for the past 15 years, and subsequently the productivity did not drop even though I served as chair/chief of a large department from 2006 to 2016

the stage of conception, others are in press. The screenshot of the Excel spreadsheet with the active projects is included below as an example. However, you can see how a stream of papers is coming along, which allows for a steady publication rate. Since 2003, there was an average of 15 papers per year (Fig. 9.5). Figure 9.6 gives an example of the current projects and their respective stages.

You want to keep things moving and zoom out from time to time to think strategically. All too often you derail, maybe because another student shows up and wants a project or because something urgent, but not important, came up. Spending time to plan your work is Quadrant 2 work! We already discussed the importance of working in the quadrant that represents important, but not urgent, work.

	A	B	C	D	E	F	G	H
1	Ongoing Projects							
2	Project No	Name	Collaborators	Collaborator Institution	Learner	Learner Status	Status	Latest update
3	1	Case report Galloway Mowat Syndrome with massive urolithiasis	Wang, Dave	UWO	N/A	N/A	Conception	Surgery performed, we have the necessary documentation - begin writing case report
4	2	Get NIH grant for hair samples in CKID study	Kaskel	Montefiori Medical	N/A	N/A	Grant funding applied	Requires revision
5	3	Long-term outcomes of childhood renal diseases	Parekh	SickKids	N/A	N/A	Grant funding applied	CIHR grant revised and submitted
6	4	FGF23 as clinical routine CRSG	Knauer	UWO	N/A	N/A	Grant funding applied	Grant submitted and not approved
7	5	Aortic Dilation Study	Grattan	UWO	Surak	PGY3	Recruitment	Lawson Approval, ready to go
8	6	Kidney stone incidence study	Ni, Lee	UWO	Ni, Lee	UGE	Recruitment	Ethics Amendments approved, also Lawson, could write the first paper of 94 patients, needs further years back - contact Vipin
9	7	ChildNeph Study	Samuel	UCalgary	N/A	N/A	Recruitment	5 additional patients have been recruited and data were entered
10	8	Telemedicine Attitudes	McIntyre	UWO	Wile	UGE	Recruitment	Recruitment slow, 5 interviews, 3 pending
11	9	UTIs in infants <35 weeks	Adie	WRH	N/A	N/A	Recruitment	Windsor is collecting additional data, needs to be rewritten
12	10	Utility of MPA monitoring in SRNS	Sharma	UWO	Kirpalani	PGY3	Rewrite manuscript, was rejected by Clin Biochem	Dose-normalized MPA and CI/F calculated, needs to focus only on enhanced clearance with nephrotic syndrome
13	11	Hepatic blood flow during HD	Huang	UWO	Grant	postgraduate	Rewrite manuscript, was rejected by NDT	Being revised
14	12	Aortic Dilation Case Report	Altamirano-Diaz	UWO	N/A	N/A	Manuscript writing, awaiting model from Sanjay Kharche	First draft written, get more details of the case, work for next week
15	13	Urinary citrate in relationship to other minerals	Bhayana	UWO	Lee	UGE	Manuscript writing	Ethics approved, calculations were performed, could begin manuscript writing
16	14	CF study	Price	UWO	Wallace	PGY2	Submitted to BMC Nephrology	Address formatting issues raised by editorial staff
17	15	Transition eGFR measurement	Ferris	UNC	Webster-Clark	UGE	Address reviewers' concerns	Awaiting the conversion factor from Maria Ferris, otherwise ready to go
18	16	Practice point POTS case	Rothfels	UWO	Rothfels	UGE	Revisions pending	Need to finalize revisions
19	17	PICCOLO MONDO world HD study	Ferris	UNC	N/A	N/A	In press	Just need to review the galley proof
20								

FIGURE 9.6 Stage of current projects, as a simple Excel spreadsheet, with titles, collaborators, learners (if applicable), learner status, status, and last update. This is updated once weekly. The darker the red, the earlier the project, the greener, the further along

Making Lists

For a more detailed to-do list, you need a program that is web-based where you can invite your collaborators. You also need to be able to assign tasks. I use MeisterTask, which is a free program that even works on your smartphone. It looks something like this (Fig. 9.7):

You have projects with various steps. The program interfaces with all of your collaborators, regardless of where they are in the world. You can detail the tasks and set due dates which will be visible to anyone who is monitoring the task. Below is one example of a project that has been submitted to NDT and has now been rejected and requires rewriting. You

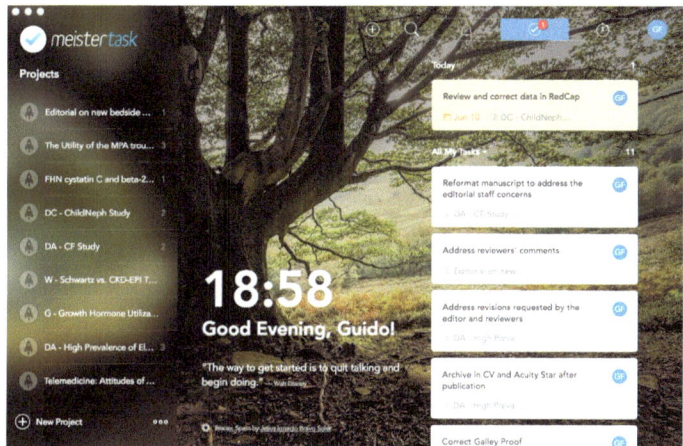

FIGURE 9.7 MeisterTask allows you to organize multiple project boards and view your main tasks on the main page

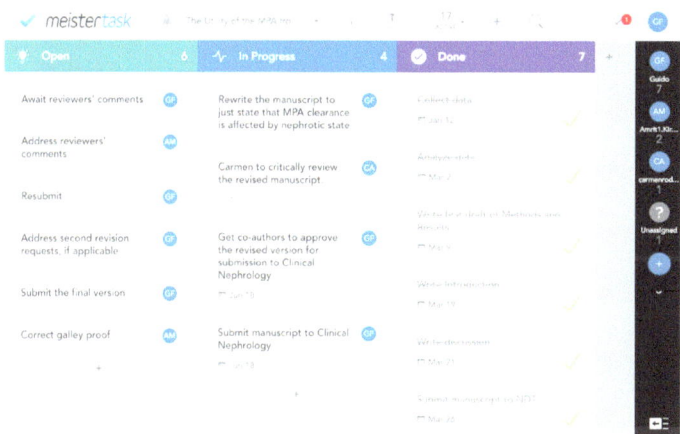

FIGURE 9.8 An example of a specific project with tasks that can further be subdivided into categories to mark your progress

can outline all steps in the beginning, move them over to "In Progress" once appropriate, and then once again move them over to "Done." The program even gives you statistics of your work (Fig. 9.8).

References

1. https://en.wikipedia.org/wiki/Robert_Cialdini.
2. Harvey SA, Wandersee JR. Publication rate of abstracts of papers and posters presented at Medical Library Association annual meetings. J Med Libr Assoc. 2010;98(3):250–5. https://doi.org/10.3163/1536-5050.98.3.014.
3. Mlinarić A, Horvat M, Šupak Smolčić V. Dealing with the positive publication bias: why you should really publish your negative results. Biochem Med (Zagreb). 2017;27(3):030201. https://doi.org/10.11613/BM.2017.030201. Review.

Chapter 10
Writing Your Paper

Literature Search and Organization

I use EndNote X8 for that task. There are free ones as well, but I have grown so used to EndNote that I do not want to learn another program. Essentially, it is a database with very useful features that enables the insertion of references in the desired format as required by the various scientific journals. Not only can you use the elegant "cite-while-you-write" feature and insert the references at the statement that you want to reference, but you can also easily format this for a specific journal, and if rejected, you can change it to a different journal style with the click of a button. It rides over Word and actually creates a new tab within the Word toolbar. On the left, you have "Insert Citation," and you just need to type in a few keywords to find it. It looks like the toolbar below (Fig. 10.1).

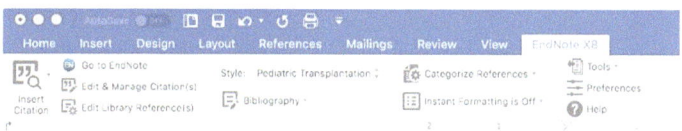

FIGURE 10.1 The toolbar display that appears once you install EndNote allows you to easily manage your citations within your Word document

© Springer Nature Switzerland AG 2019
G. Filler, R. Nagra, *Becoming a Successful Scholar*,
https://doi.org/10.1007/978-3-030-24448-4_10

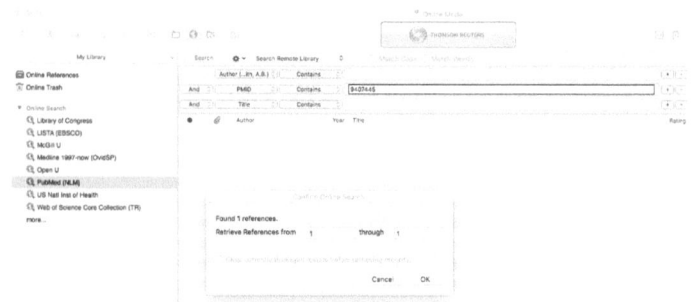

FIGURE 10.2 Searching up the PubMedID allows you to directly retrieve and import the citation

You can also store the actual PDFs of the papers in the database for quick reference, and the abstracts are included in the database. You can import the references from various sources. Personally, I use PubMed and just import using the PubMed ID. Importing the reference rather than typing it in will reduce inevitable errors in your citations (Fig. 10.2).

You can download a plethora of journal styles to format your references accordingly (Fig. 10.3).

Journal reviewers and editors do not take kindly to wrong references, so you want to get this 100% right. You also want to avoid messing up your references if you use them more than once, or if you change the order of your manuscript's text around, the numbering must remain consistent.

If you need to reformat the references for another journal, it will just take the click of a button. Furthermore, you want only one library for each project, and you want it "in the clouds" so that you can access it wherever you are in order to write. Right now, for instance, I am flying from Toronto to México City, and such time is perfect for working on your projects as there is absolutely nothing to do during this 4.5-hour flight, other than perhaps playing some mindless games on your phone or watching a movie. I had some difficulties with the cloud databases when I upgraded to EndNote X8, and another option you have is to have your database on platforms such as Google Drive or Dropbox so that you can access it from anywhere. This avoids the synchronization

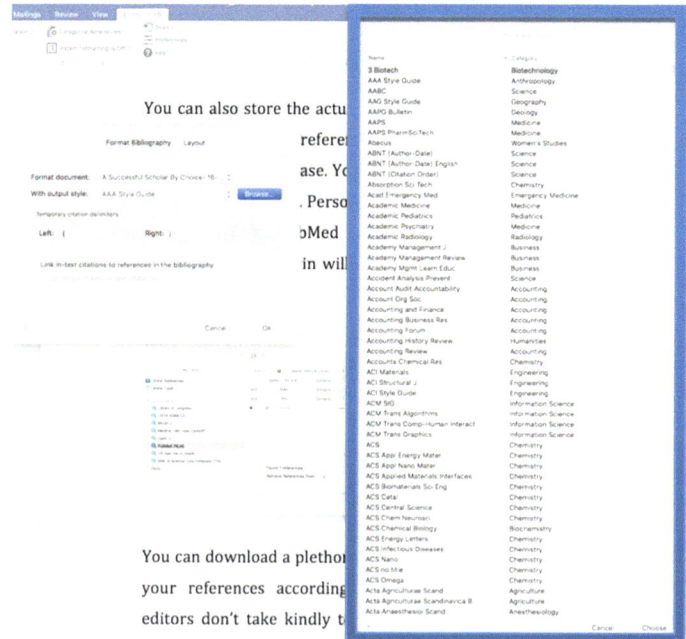

FIGURE 10.3 A snippet of the various journal styles that you may choose from for your specific paper

issues; however, you will have to close EndNote at all times when switching from one device to another. The cloud synchronization is probably the best approach. All of this can be achieved with commercial programs such as EndNote X8, which rides on top of Word, almost invisible. There are alternatives, such as Reference Manager, or Mendeley, which is free.

Organizing Your Work: Literature Search

Now schedule 1 hour each day, let us say, for 1 week, to develop a thorough database for your paper. For that 1 hour, assign the task of collecting eight to ten relevant references. You may wish to use the proxy server of your university library for that task so that you can download the PDFs. If the library does not have access to your particular journal of choice, you may consider some "illegal" pirate tools to get the PDFs instead, but of course, I should discourage that. As a resourceful future researcher, I am sure you will find this information. Professional social media platforms that allow self-archiving, such as ResearchGate which is also free, may be a good alternative for obtaining PDFs of papers that you want to read and use. Most journals allow some form of self-archiving, and you can store your precious reprints online and share them privately upon request. More and more researchers make a profile on ResearchGate, and I am actually getting inundated with the requests on there.

For the literature search, I use PubMed, which is free and very complete. Some folks say, if a reference is not indexed on PubMed, it is likely from a predatory journal, and not to use such a citation. I try to use only references that are indexed in PubMed. This also avoids manual entries of references into EndNote. Errors with citations are quite embarrassing when you have to address them after peer review or, worse, after publication. Importing eight to ten references and uploading the PDFs will take you 5 minutes per reference max. I would also recommend that you keep a Word document open to write a brief summary of each paper that you choose to include in your database. This summary should be no more than three sentences highlighting the main thought or teaching of the manuscript. Having a good database with references is always the very first step for any paper. I ask any learner whom I supervise to start with that task. Over 1 week, you will have at least 56 references, which is a good start. I also recommend that you structure your summary Word document with a table of contents and organize the references you have obtained in themes. This is actually how I write reviews as well; the structured Word document is incredibly helpful. Ideally, you do this in a separate database program, and not in Word, so that you can organize your references even better, but cut and paste works just fine for the organization for me, and you do not need to have yet another program open.

Organizing Your Work: Formatting Your Manuscript

After 1 week, if you follow the outlined suggestions, you should have your database. Now, you want to write the introduction. Before you go ahead, let us just *zoom out* for a second for some important considerations.

Formatting of manuscripts varies by journal, and you need to read and ideally print the instructions for authors of your journal of choice and follow them to the "t." It can be quite confusing to find the relevant information, and often it is incomplete. Fortunately, more and more journals are embracing a standardization of reporting. This really helps to improve the quality and consistency of reporting. The most advanced approach is the CONSORT (*Con*solidated *S*tandards *of Reporting Trials*) statement. The CONSORT statement was developed by scientists working with David Moher from the University of Ottawa for the reporting of randomized controlled clinical trials. Soon thereafter, other statements were developed for other types of studies. For instance, a cross-sectional epidemiological study would follow the STROBE (*St*rengthening the *R*eporting of *OB*servational studies in *E*pidemiology) statement. Your one-stop shop for any study type is the EQUATOR (*E*nhancing the *QUA*lity and *T*ransparency *o*f Health *R*esearch) statement, which links you to any study type. I would recommend that you develop any publication using the appropriate structures from the EQUATOR website and also download the appropriate checklists and submit the completed checklist together with each manuscript, regardless of whether the journal endorses the EQUATOR statement or not (Fig. 10.4). There is nothing missing when you do so, and you can easily reformat from one journal to another if the manuscript is rejected.

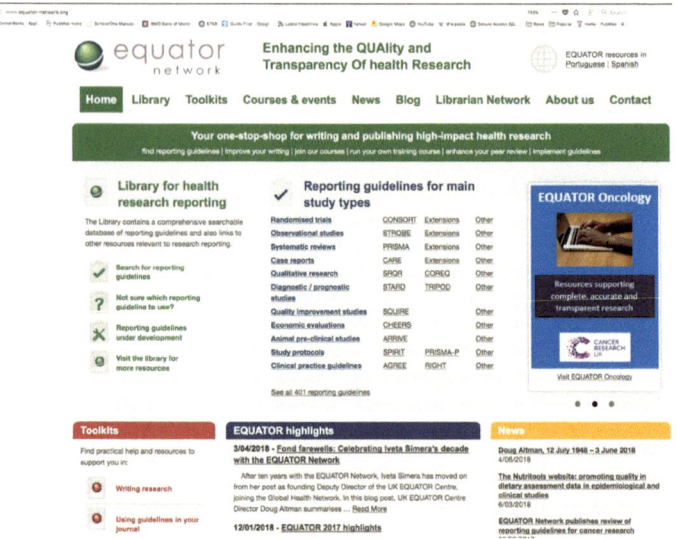

FIGURE 10.4 EQUATOR's checklists are available for download on their website based on your study type

EQUATOR is a network that attempts to actively involve multiple stakeholders across the globe and bring together researchers, editors, and reviewers to produce comprehensive guidelines for reporting research publications. Research results increase their own value and significance in the scientific world by being replicable and available to the public. This is the foundation of modern research. Ensuring protocols and experimental setups are available and clearly communicated allows the validity of the research to be established. The EQUATOR Network has several primary goals that is attempting to achieve transparent and accurate reporting such as:

- Providing an online resource with current materials and tools that are relevant for research reporting within the health field.
- Promoting the use of research reporting guidelines and completing education and training programs.

- Setting up global EQUATOR centers so that research reporting reaches a high standard that is consistently followed.

- Encouraging universities, journals, and other educative faculties to endorse and implement reporting guidelines.

By striving to achieve these goals and by having various corporations and editors approve of their methods, EQATOR increases the ability of available research evidence to have increasing usability and relevance in the scientific and public sphere. Unfortunately, most universities do not teach about EQUATOR.org, even though the skill to assess the quality of a publication is essential for any scholar or, in fact, any professional. Checking a manuscript using one of their checklists is actually a really good way to assess the quality by simply checking adherence to each aspect.

When we last looked at the journal list that endorsed the EQUATOR statement, there were 177 journals listed (http://www.equator-network.org/about-us/organisations-supporting-equator/, accessed 14-Jun-2018). EQUATOR conveniently has a link for the reporting guidelines that should be used for various types of studies with a simplified and easy-to-follow Word document available for each reporting guideline, allowing you to produce a paper to the highest reporting standard. There are various types of manuscripts available to choose from to obtain a reporting guideline checklist. For instance, randomized trials (CONSORT guidelines), observational studies (STROBE), systematic reviews (PRISMA – *P*referred *R*eporting *I*tems for *S*ystematic Reviews and *M*eta-*A*nalyses), case reports (CARE – *CA*se *Re*port), Qualitative research (SRQR or COREQ), diagnostic or prognostic studies (STARD or TRIPOD), quality improvement studies (SQUIRE), economic evaluations (CHEERS), animal preclinical studies (ARRIVE), study protocols (SPIRIT or PRISMA-P), and clinical practice guidelines (AGREE or RIGHT) all have their own checklists.

Let us assume you have conducted a cross-sectional study. This would be most appropriate for the STROBE statement. To illustrate how you go forward, I will focus on the STROBE checklist for cross-sectional studies (see Table 10.1 below).

TABLE 10.1 STROBE statement – checklist of items that should be included in reports of *cross-sectional studies*

	Item no	Recommendation
Title and abstract	1	(a) Indicate the study's design with a commonly used term in the title or the abstract
		(b) Provide in the abstract an informative and balanced summary of what was done and what was found
Introduction		
Background/ rationale	2	Explain the scientific background and rationale for the investigation being reported
Objectives	3	State specific objectives, including any prespecified hypotheses
Methods		
Study design	4	Present key elements of study design early in the paper
Setting	5	Describe the setting, locations, and relevant dates, including periods of recruitment, exposure, follow-up, and data collection
Participants	6	(a) Give the eligibility criteria, and the sources and methods of selection of participants
Variables	7	Clearly define all outcomes, exposures, predictors, potential confounders, and effect modifiers. Give diagnostic criteria, if applicable
Data sources/ measurement	8[a]	For each variable of interest, give sources of data and details of methods of assessment (measurement). Describe comparability of assessment methods if there is more than one group

Bias	9	Describe any efforts to address potential sources of bias
Study size	10	Explain how the study size was arrived at
Quantitative variables	11	Explain how quantitative variables were handled in the analyses. If applicable, describe which groupings were chosen and why
Statistical methods	12	(a) Describe all statistical methods, including those used to control for confounding
		(b) Describe any methods used to examine subgroups and interactions
		(c) Explain how missing data were addressed
		(d) If applicable, describe analytical methods taking account of sampling strategy
		(e) Describe any sensitivity analyses
Results		
Participants	13[a]	(a) Report numbers of individuals at each stage of study – e.g., numbers potentially eligible, examined for eligibility, confirmed eligible, included in the study, completing follow-up, and analyzed
		(b) Give reasons for non-participation at each stage
		(c) Consider use of a flow diagram

(continued)

TABLE 10.1 (continued)

	Item no	Recommendation
Descriptive data	14[a]	(a) Give characteristics of study participants (e.g., demographic, clinical, social) and information on exposures and potential confounders
		(b) Indicate number of participants with missing data for each variable of interest
Outcome data	15[a]	Report numbers of outcome events or summary measures
Main results	16	(a) Give unadjusted estimates and, if applicable, confounder-adjusted estimates and their precision (e.g., 95% confidence interval). Make clear which confounders were adjusted for and why they were included
		(b) Report category boundaries when continuous variables were categorized
		(c) If relevant, consider translating estimates of relative risk into absolute risk for a meaningful time period
Other analyses	17	Report other analyses done – e.g., analyses of subgroups and interactions, and sensitivity analyses
Discussion		
Key results	18	Summarize key results with reference to study objectives

Limitations	19	Discuss limitations of the study, taking into account sources of potential bias or imprecision. Discuss both direction and magnitude of any potential bias
Interpretation	20	Give a cautious overall interpretation of results considering objectives, limitations, multiplicity of analyses, results from similar studies, and other relevant evidence
Generalizability	21	Discuss the generalizability (external validity) of the study results
Other information		
Funding	22	Give the source of funding and the role of the funders for the present study and, if applicable, for the original study on which the present article is based

Note: An Explanation and Elaboration article discusses each checklist item and gives methodological background and published examples of transparent reporting. The STROBE checklist is best used in conjunction with this article (freely available on the Web sites of PLoS Medicine at http://www.plosmedicine.org/, Annals of Internal Medicine at http://www.annals.org/, and Epidemiology at http://www.epidem.com/). Information on the STROBE Initiative is available at www.strobe-statement.org

[a]Give information separately for exposed and unexposed groups

Once you have figured out the proper formatting guidelines you will be following, you should schedule time for writing the introduction.

Before You Start Writing

Journals (and their editors) seek original articles that are novel, important, informative, and ethical. They only want to see papers that are free of commercial or intellectual bias. It is important in the digital age that work is timely and adherent to principles of trial registration and conduct (see EQUATOR statement).

Please note that a lot of the organization of your paper has already been set by your research beforehand. Many things that you have described in the ethics approval and grant will be reflected in the paper. For instance, the problem to be studied and the hypothesis belong in the introduction. How you carried out the experiments belongs in materials and methods. The results will go to the results section, and the interpretation will go into the discussion and conclusion. One way to plan a paper is to do it visually, just like you would map out a poster. An example is given below (Fig. 10.5).

When you prepare a poster, you already have half of your paper done. You have the same structural elements as the paper; however, it is obviously much shorter.

Choosing the Journal

You want to write an important paper. You want to consider the right audience. In order to write an important paper, the information you want to convey needs to add appreciably, not just incrementally. The conclusions, or the teachable moment, must provide clear direction. People focus a lot on impact factor and journal prestige when choosing a journal. However, if your teachable moment is to target a pediatric nephrology

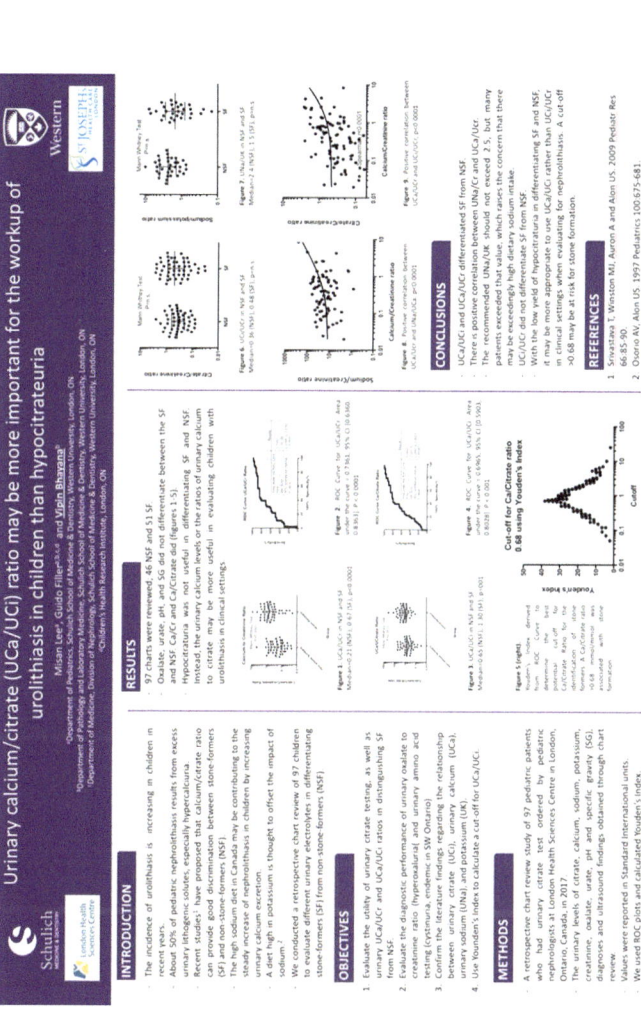

FIGURE 10.5 This poster presentation on our retrospective study allowed all the information to be clearly divided into the separate sections and is able to be used as a template for the actual paper

audience, the most widely read journal is *Pediatric Nephrology*. So if your findings substantially and appreciably increment the knowledge of what is important to a pediatric nephrologist, then target that journal. The impact factor is increasingly important for the institutions because they are all in competition with each other, but I believe you should instead focus on the appropriate target audience.

Take a minute to reflect and really ask yourself the question; does your paper fit the aims and scope of the journal? Read the scope of the journal section. Issues you want to consider are what percentage of submissions are accepted by how is the journal viewed, and what is their speed of publishing? If you have something very important that needs to be published, let us say about peritoneal dialysis, then *Peritoneal Dialysis International*, which is published quarterly and has a slow review process, may not be the most appropriate journal. By contrast, you have a particular finding, for instance, the age dependency of icodextrin clearance in children; then this journal would be by far the most appropriate journal. These are all important issues when deciding about where to submit your work.

Consider whether the journal is for a general audience, whether it is a specialty, or even sub-specialty journal. *JAMA* is a general audience journal, *Pediatrics* is a specialty journal, and *Pediatric Nephrology* is a sub-specialty journal.

The next question is what type of review is being done. You do not want to fall into the trap of predatory journals that do not perform proper peer review. There was a list online by Jeoffrey Beall that listed all predatory journals. Unfortunately, some journals started a huge fight and the list had to be taken offline. However, there are buffers, and you can still find the information through Google. *AVOID PREDATORY JOURNALS!* Publishing in these journals may actually harm your career. Predatory open-access publishing is an exploitative open-access academic publishing business model that involves charging publication fees to authors without providing the editorial and publishing services associated with legitimate journals (open access or not).

Unfortunately, the number of these predatory journals is sky-rocketing. You can identify them by the following characteristics:

- Accepting articles quickly with little or no peer review or quality control, including hoax and nonsensical papers.
- Notifying academics of article fees only after papers are accepted.
- Aggressively campaigning for academics to submit articles or serve on editorial boards.
- Listing academics as members of editorial boards without their permission, and not allowing academics to resign from editorial boards.
- Appointing fake academics to editorial boards.
- Mimicking the name or website style of more established journals.
- Making misleading claims about the publishing operation, such as a false location.
- Using ISSNs improperly.
- Citing fake or nonexistent impact factors.

List taken from: https://en.wikipedia.org/wiki/Predatory_open-access_publishing, accessed 14-Jun-2018

Another aspect is whether or not to publish in an open-access journal. In principle, an open-access journal is a good idea because the information should be in the public domain and not copyrighted by the publishers. Apart from the fleet of predatory open-access publishers, there are some very credible open-access publishers like *PLOS One* or the *BMC* series. Unfortunately, their pricing is prohibitive, usually about North of $2000 USD per paper. However, you get a high impact factor. You would only consider that if you have budgeted accordingly in your grant submission. There are a few credible, free open-access journals, such as *Clinical Kidney Journal*, which just extended the free publication for another year. This journal is owned by the European Dialysis and Transplantation Association. Unfortunately, they often do not have a high impact factor. Another credible example is the *Indian Journal of Nephrology*. Again, a society sponsored the journal.

For the most part, you will likely publish without open access. Be careful about the author's and publisher's rights are and obey them. Please note that there may still be other expenses for surplus page charges and submission charges. All of these points, as well as the journal's reputation and rank, are important for your journal decision. If the journal you wish to publish in rejects your paper, be prepared and willing to revise and resubmit elsewhere.

Writing the Introduction

Now, for your introduction, you really only need three elements, namely, background, rationale, and objectives. I usually write the introduction in just 45 minutes, but if you want, you can schedule three to four 45-minute sessions over several days. You should also state a specific hypothesis at the end of your introduction. The introduction should be concise and clear, usually not exceeding one page. Make sure you only include information that matches your study, and remember, an introduction is not meant to be a complete review of a field. State with a few sentences what is known and what knowledge gaps exist. Do not make it exhaustive.

Writing the Methods

Accurately describing your methods is essential in getting a paper published, as your results should be replicable with the exact same protocols. Make sure you clearly provide the primary and secondary aims in this section, distinct from the hypotheses. Coherently describe the study design and the data that was collected, and if necessary, include the assay details. Your methods should also be very specific in describing the subjects participating, and what the inclusion or exclusion criteria were. Lastly, the statistical tests used and the criteria for significance should be explained here. These details, while seemingly minute, are critical and must not be left out. It is not sufficient to simply refer to other publications for information regarding how your study consent was attained.

Writing the Results

You will likely have a copious amount of data collected, but it is important that you carefully select your data to reflect what is critical. Relevancy and significance are of utmost importance, and it is imperative that you do not list all numbers from tables in the text and that you do not exclude data that does not fit well with your hypotheses or expected results. Use tables and figures to summarize the data collected, including one to list subject characteristics. Within your actual text, make sure the main findings are clear, and you refer to your figures when discussing findings. Also, make sure that your methods and your results match exactly. Anything you describe in the results section has to be outlined and described in the methods section. Similarly, do not have anything in the methods section that you do not need for the results section.

Writing the Discussion

This section of your paper will allow many readers to get a better understanding of the wider applicability of your study. The first paragraph should be a simple summary of your main findings, which refers to previous work in the field and shows the relevancy of your work. Next, in a couple of paragraphs, implications that can be logically drawn from the results obtained should be addressed. Follow this with the possible limitations that were present, and if possible, refer to literature that may suggest these issues are not hindering to the overall findings. You may finish this section by summarizing the strengths of your study. Remember, ignoring or being over defensive regarding your limitations will not be viewed kindly by the reviewers! Just state the facts. Also, make sure you do not make claims of priority, such as "This is the first…" or "This is the only…". Importantly, do not use any jargon either.

All these points, along with a short and accurate summary, should be addressed in less than four pages for your discussion. This final section of your paper should accurately discuss your findings and their logical importance within the field and current literature. Consider two things: what are the implications and are your findings generalizable? Remember, do not make your focus a criticism of other studies, as those same authors might be the ones reviewing your paper for the journal!

Chapter 11
Perseverance

Collins dictionary defines perseverance as follows: "Perseverance is the quality of continuing with something even though it is difficult."

This particular character trait is so important that it is worth writing a separate chapter about it. Imagine you performed a study, presented it as an abstract, but "only" as a poster at an international conference. During the conference, folks criticized your work really hard. They stated that your assumptions were wrong and that your work was biased. Still, you decide to put this into a manuscript. You do not agree with the criticism. You sent it to a couple of high-level journals that you deemed important for the subject matter, and all rejected it quickly without a formal review. The journals thanked you for your interest, and no further reasons were disclosed. You then decided to turn to a low-ranking journal, and they actually did send it out for review. You chose the reviewers from the field, and you received a devastating rejection from the three reviewers who did not agree with the paradigm shift that you proposed. What do you do? You might as well give up!

Many of your peers feel similarly. Have you invested all your work and time in vain? Before digging into how to persevere through rejection and why it is a characteristic of utmost importance, it is essential to discuss why your work

© Springer Nature Switzerland AG 2019   109
G. Filler, R. Nagra, *Becoming a Successful Scholar*,
https://doi.org/10.1007/978-3-030-24448-4_11

can get rejected and look a little more into the logistics publications. For a start, it is essential that you remember that not everything that is presented should be published. While abstracts presented in meetings actually have a significant effect on decision-making and medical practice, one needs to be aware of considerable bias. Considerable pressure is placed on rapid dissemination of response data in clinical trials. Yet, initial response rates may not reflect the true behavior of intervention as outcomes may change with time and may not be mature for several years. Published abstracts often over- or underestimate the initial response rate to an intervention [1]. So it may not always be desirable to prematurely publish results.

Beyond this issue, the overall rate of published full articles is usually only about 25%. In a study of the poster and oral abstracts at the American College of Cardiology 58th Annual Scientific Session 2009, between 24% and 30% of posters achieved a full publication by October 2012, i.e., 3 years after the conference [2]. In some sessions, the publication rate was as low as 6%, for instance, in "quality of care" and "outcomes" sessions.

Data on the percentage of research projects that do not even get to a presentation at an international conference are difficult to come by, but it is expected to be a considerable amount.

It is well known that there are large differences in the publication output between scientists. Only a relatively small proportion of scientists contribute to the majority of publications. In 1926, Lotka formulated the famous inverse square law of productivity, which states that the number of authors producing n papers is approximately $1/n^2$ of those producing one [3]. This means that of all authors in a given field, some 60% will have produced just one publication. Many other researchers have subsequently confirmed this very skewed publication record.

What do we know about the reasons for the low publication rates? Several studies have considered the impact of gender, age, and academic position of the researchers.

However, in a study of 12,400 Norwegian university research-ers, the research team showed that age and gender were not important, only the academic position was [4]. These findings are not surprising. It is conceivable that professors will have the highest publication rates, as they achieve their career's success based on publications. The junior personnel are less experienced as researchers. As knowledge is cumulative, a scientist in a senior position is more likely to have better abilities to do research and write articles. Moreover, senior personnel often have lead roles in the research process and may be involved in many research projects at the same time, resulting in more publications.

Another aspect that always came out in studies was on the impact of gender. Many studies have shown that female sci-entists tend to publish fewer publications than their male colleagues. However, usually, the proportion of female researchers decreases within the hierarchy of positions. The issue that historically more men were in senior positions is complex. As the population demographics of females in aca-demic positions continues to change, I believe it is just a mat-ter of time until both genders will be equally represented at each level. When you do compare men and women in similar career stages even today, there was no difference in academic success.

Furthermore, the relationship between age and publica-tion rate has been found to be curvilinear in several studies. The average production of publications increases with age and reaches a peak at some point during the career before it declines. It should be pointed out that researchers with more recognition keep publishing frequently after their less-recog-nized peers have reached their zenith. It should also be pointed out that women may reach their zenith much later owing to the natural break during childbearing age, and often surpassing males in their 60s and 70s.

The study by Rørstad and Aksnes determined that most of the variance cannot be explained by the factors named above, and they conclude their manuscript by stating that "publication rate also depends on a wide range of factors that cannot easily be measured, such as: the availability of research funds; teaching loads; equipment; research assistants; workload policies; departmental culture and working conditions; organizational context; and talent and hard work." Moreover, they write "the process of cumulative advantage implies that minor differences early in a career may result in substantial differences in achievement by the end of a career. Success in scientific careers may depend on the ability of the scientists themselves but also on luck (cf. the distinction between virtu and fortuna by Turner & Chubin, 1979)." We already talked about luck, and I dare to disagree by saying it depends on the return on luck, not on luck. Working well above the death line may account for what was said for differences early in the career, and fanatic discipline may well be the difference in the talent. However, I think what is most important is perseverance!

What do I mean by that? Consider a rejected paper. Your first reaction is anger and disbelief. You disregard the fact that some journals may simply reject papers on priority grounds and that some journals may have acceptance rates as low as 10%. In the summary report of journal operations of 2016, the average rejection rate of psychological journals was 71% [5]. You experience pain and blame yourself, you have not worked hard enough. Then reality hits, and you continue to read the comments made by the reviewers. You are now in shock and denial. Eventually, you show this to friends, colleagues, or co-authors, and you start to debate with them about the reasons behind some comments, as well as voicing your ifs and whens and buts. A state of depression often follows this. It is almost like the seven stages of grief:

- Shock and denial
- Pain and guilt
- Anger and bargaining
- Depression, reflection, loneliness
- The upward turn
- Reconstruction and working through
- Acceptance and hope

I believe that all too often, young researchers get stuck in phase 4, namely, depression, reflection, and loneliness. I propose that instead, researchers should see failure and rejection as an opportunity and try to get to phase 7: acceptance and hope quickly.

What should you do to get there? The first and foremost advice is to read what the reviewer said, ideally without emotion carefully. Do not just dismiss their comments. Make an itemized list with every point, similar to what you would do if you address minor or major revisions of a manuscript that was not rejected. Then systematically work yourself through every single point, with repeating the statement, an answer or rebuttal to each point, and suggested changes to the manuscript. I do this regardless whether a manuscript was asked to be revised or whether it was rejected. To just reformat the manuscript and to submit it to another journal is only wise if the paper was merely rejected on priority grounds in a high-ranking journal. Never ignore the reviewers' comments, and do not dismiss them by thinking "they did not understand" or "they are biased." You will lose significant opportunities with this attitude. Usually, reviewers' views reflect the mainstream reasoning, and you may not get beyond them if you ignore this. Rather, consider each point with respect and modesty. Word your rebuttal of a contentious point with calm and reason, and try to use maximum clarity in your response. It will help you to see with clarity how you can overcome the biases or preconceptions, especially when you break with a paradigm.

I also recommend that you use *Track Changes* in Word when you revise your manuscript and that you work one step at a time. Every journey begins with one step, and similarly, you need to consider one point at a time. Schedule this work so that it does not become exhaustive or tedious. Maybe you want to work on the comments of only one reviewer at a time for a session. You will need a deep level of concentration for this work. If you have 3 reviewers and each has 10–15 points to be addressed, you cannot afford to address them all at once, because your concentration will decline, as well as the quality of your work.

If you do this systematically, you will eventually get the paper published. I want to give you an example, which is something that I am actually rather proud of. During my tenure as chair/chief, a few years ago, I wanted to answer the question of whether the variability of the physician specialist supply actually affects health outcomes. The question about the "why does this matter?" was easy to answer: If we could demonstrate this link, we could use this as a powerful argument to request more specialist and subspecialists in the academic centers to improve outcomes to a desirable level. However, this was not an easy question to address. It has been shown by many that physician access varies substantially across a country. In Canada, we have high supply provinces for pediatricians and pediatric subspecialists (measured as specialists or subspecialists per 100,000 population) such as Newfoundland, Manitoba, and Alberta. By contrast, Saskatchewan, British Columbia, and Ontario are low supply territories. In the United States, the variability may be even greater. In Fig. 11.1, you can see the

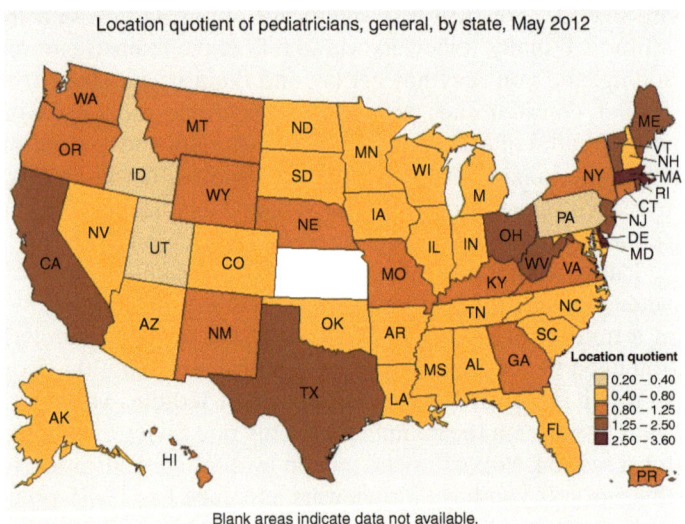

FIGURE 11.1 Location quotient of pediatricians, by state, in May of 2012. (Data are from http://www.bls.gov/oes/current/oes291065. htm#nat)

location quotient of pediatricians by state in 2012. As can easily be seen, there is a more than 15-fold variability between low supply states, such as Idaho, and high supply states, such as Delaware or Massachusetts.

In Canada, the Paediatric Chairs of Canada (PCC), together with the Canadian Institute of Health Information (CIHI), was able to generate maps of all the available providers of healthcare for children and youth across the country. The size of the triangles reflects the ratio of either generalist, specialists, or subspecialists per 100,000 children. Please see Fig. 11.2. The data is expressed as physicians per dissemination area.

Particular focus should be paid to the fact that large rural communities have no access to pediatricians at all. Together with Dr. Leonard Huang from McMaster, I was fortunate to lead the physician workforce project of the Paediatric Chairs of Canada.

There are many reasons for this, some may have to do with the geographic realities, but as a general rule, the community-based specialists often settle close to their "alma mater," while subspecialists may require a tertiary care institution to conduct their work. For instance, it would be impossible for pediatric nephrologists to perform dialysis treatments anywhere outside of a larger dialysis center in an academic center.

For our study's questions, we decided to perform a pilot project and focus on asthma admissions, the severity of the cases, and lengths of stay as well as readmission rates among similar regional health authorities in Manitoba and Saskatchewan [6]. This was largely done because the climate, growing season length, pollen exposure, and other well-known factors for childhood asthma are pretty similar in both prairie states. The variability of physician supply was vastly different (Fig. 11.3).

We then had to come up with a methodology to compare regions with similar environmental, socioeconomic, and demographic factors that influence disease prevalence, to ensure that we were comparing "apples with apples" and not

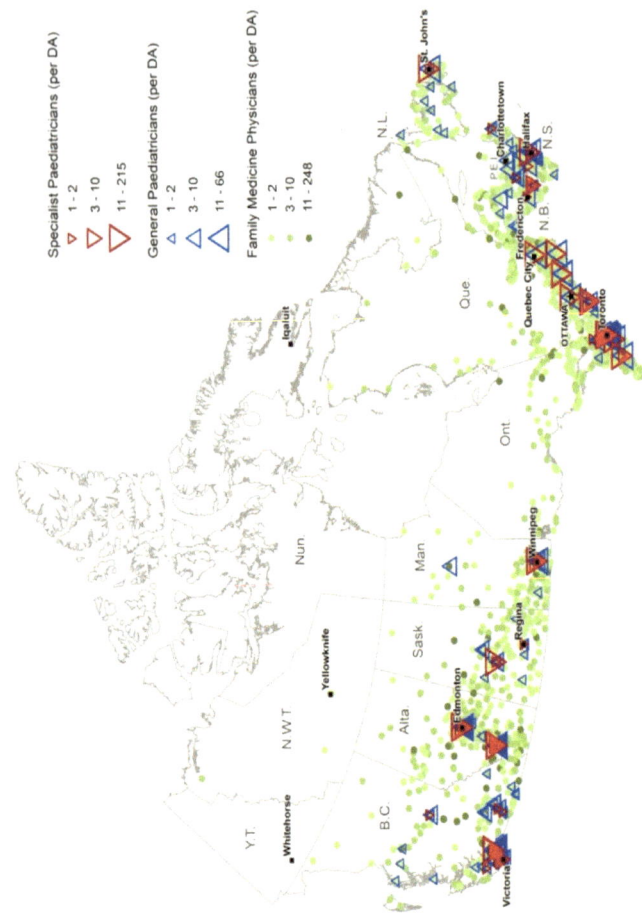

FIGURE 11.2
Distribution of family medicine physicians, general pediatricians, and specialist pediatricians in Canada per Dissemination Area, 2011. (Unpublished work and courtesy of the Paediatric Chairs of Canada and CIHI, based on data from Scott's Medical Database 2014, CIHI, and the Paediatric Chairs of Canada)

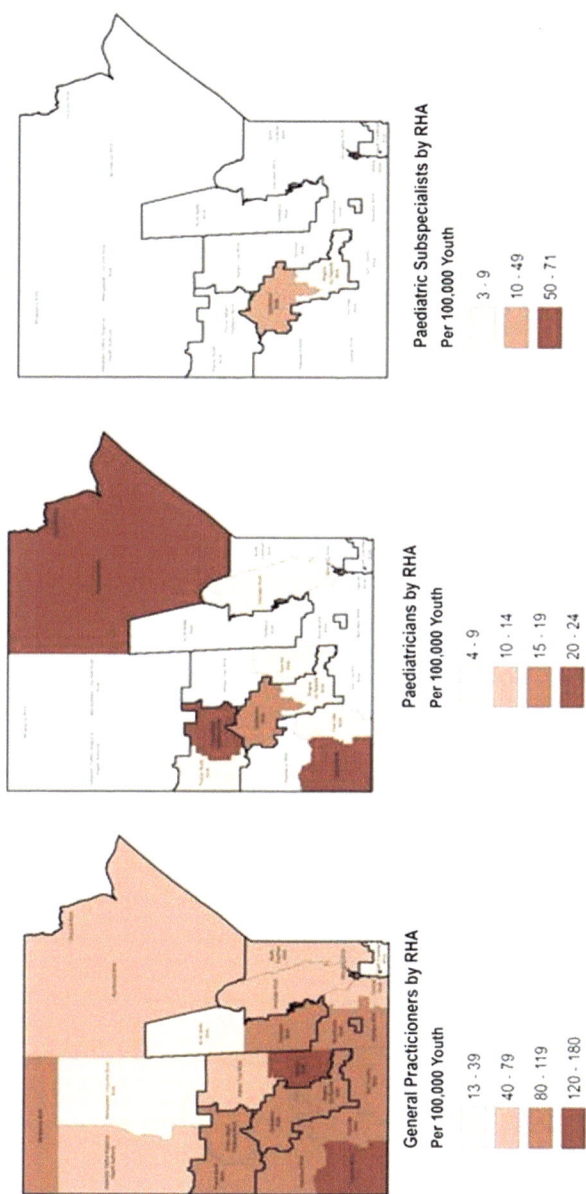

FIGURE 11.3 Distribution of general practitioners, pediatricians, and pediatric subspecialists by regional health authority (RHA), color coded by density

"oranges." With the help of Eric Bourdon from CIHI, we decided to use peer group Regional Health Authorities (RHA), which are based on similar populations, locations, socioeconomic status, and other factors. When comparing the asthma admission rates by similar peer group RHAs, we found amazing differences that were directly related to access to specialists and subspecialists. At the provincial level, Manitoba had 48.6 pediatricians/100,000 child population, compared to 23.5/100,000 in Saskatchewan. As for pediatric asthma specialists, in Manitoba, there were 3.1/100,000 child population and 1.4/100,000 in Saskatchewan. Among peer group A, the differences were even more striking. A significantly higher number of patients were admitted in Saskatchewan (590.3/100,000 children) compared to Manitoba (309.3/100,000, p <0.0001). Saskatchewan, which has a lower pediatrician and pediatric asthma specialist supply, had a higher asthma admission rate than Manitoba. Our data suggest that there is an inverse relationship between asthma admissions and pediatrician and asthma specialist supply.

You could evidently argue that this information is important, and it certainly helped my colleague in Saskatoon to successfully advocate for a significant number of new pediatric pulmonology positions. Publication of this manuscript, however, proved to be exceedingly difficult. I should point out that this piece of work was rather translational, with many authors with very different skills and fields of work were involved, including health geographers, members of the Canadian Institute of Health Information, the president and CEO of the Canadian Association of Paediatric Health Centres, as well as physician subspecialists and department chairs.

We first sent the manuscript to a couple of asthma journals. They rejected it based on insufficient control of confounders of the prevalence of childhood asthma. Then we moved on the *Canadian Medical Association Journal Open* (CMAJ Open) because of the implications for the nationwide health human research planning. In their decision letter, it states: "Although your topic is an interesting one, I am sorry to tell you that we have decided to decline your manuscript for publication. The editors at *CMAJ Open* who carefully read your manuscript decided that the study design and analytic approach is inadequate given the question you were trying to answer. It is unfortunate that a multivariate analysis was not possible due to privacy regulations. As a result, the findings represent too minor an increment in knowledge to be considered for publication in the *CMAJ Open*." With a comment telling us our hard work amounted to "too minor an increment in knowledge," we might as well have given up! But we did not!

We were afraid that the *CMAJ* did not understand the complexity of the analysis and sent it to the *Lancet* because we felt they might appreciate the novelty of the approach. The *Lancet* rejected on priority grounds. We then sent the manuscript to a health geography journal, and we applied for a grant to get a more extensive study off the ground. This was also rejected, as there was not enough health geography. Another attempt at *EBioMedicine*. Rejected. The next submission was to *Human Resources for Health*. They were more favorable but requested major revisions that were difficult to address. I confess that there was an element of depression kicking in because so much energy had gone into this work and I really wanted to continue on this path. The work demonstrated a link between specialist and subspecialist supply: the health outcomes could be used to determine the health resources needed for Canada based on a comparison of admission rates and length of stay compared to the expected length of stay. I must also confess that I parked the manuscript for 2 years because I became swamped with the end of my second term as chair/chief of the department and the newly acquired role as vice chair of the Medical Advisory Committee. Eventually, I opted for *BMC Health Services* research. It took three revisions to get it accepted finally.

Each time, we incorporated the reviewer comments. What is fascinating is the fact that every journal had different grounds on which they had rejected the manuscript. It was my friend William Smoyer, MD, who is a member of the Section of Nephrology at Nationwide Children's Hospital, Vice President and Director for the Center for Clinical and Translational Research at The Research Institute at Nationwide Children's Hospital, who debunked this seemingly random pattern for me. He stated that the fate of his first truly translational paper was very similar. Each speciality or subspecialty journal has a particular viewpoint. There is a paucity of translational research journals that fully acknowledge the challenges of being 100% attuned to each aspect of the translational work.

Without a doubt, it does help immensely to see the reviewers' and editors' perspectives. Perhaps the most enabling aspect of my success as an author has been me exercising the role of a reviewer and editor. Ideally, you need to write the paper as if you see it from the reviewer's and editor's perspective.

It should be your goal to get at least 90% of your abstracts published as full papers. Why would you want to invest all the work and not bear the fruit? Brace for the challenges that may intimidate you and see them as opportunities. Anticipate rejection. Have backup plans and quickly return to the "acceptance and hope" stage of grief. Ask yourself if your last version of your paper *really* is the best you can do? Compete with yourself! Of course, all the behaviors stated before (like fanatic discipline and fire bullets, *then* cannonballs) are also really important, but in my humble opinion, perseverance is the most important character trait you can possess for you to become an accomplished scholar.

References

1. Beyar-Katz O, Rowe JM, Townsend LE, Tallman MS, Hadomi R, Horowitz NA. Published abstracts at international meetings often over- or underestimate the initial response rate. Blood. 2017;129:2326–8. https://doi.org/10.1182/blood-2017-01-763144.
2. Percentage of poster and oral abstracts at the American College of Cardiology 58th annual scientific session 2009 that achieved publication with their journal impact factors. https://doi.org/10.1016/j.ijcard.2013.01.237.

3. Lotka AJ. The frequency distribution of scientific productivity. J Wash Acad Sci. 1926;16(12):317–23.
4. Kristoffer Rørstad Dag W. Aksnes. Publication rate expressed by age, gender and academic position – a large-scale analysis of Norwegian academic staff. https://doi.org/10.1016/j.joi.2015.02.003.
5. http://www.apa.org/pubs/journals/features/2016-statistics.pdf.
6. Filler G, Kovesi T, Bourdon E, Jones SA, et al. Does specialist physician supply affect pediatric asthma health outcomes? BMC Health Serv Res. 2018;18(1):247. https://doi.org/10.1186/s12913-018-3084-z.

Chapter 12
Reviewing

Nick Feamster: Learning how to review papers not only (obviously) makes you a better reviewer, but it can also help you as an author, since an understanding of the process can help you write your paper submissions for an audience of reviewers. If you know the criteria that a reviewer will use to judge your paper, you are in a much better position to tailor your paper so that it has a higher chance of being accepted. [1]

One of the best strategies for becoming a better author is to become a great reviewer. There are many resources that teach you how to become a better reviewer. We already talked about the EQUATOR statement and how to find a mature template and checklist for any type of scientific paper. You need to understand the review process. Not only is knowing the process a great tool for helping you write better papers suited to the audience of reviewers, but it also helps you to understand why a paper is accepted or rejected, and from the last paper, we know rejection rates are high and should not deter you from your goals.

As a senior author who has published a lot in the field of pediatric renal transplantation or measurement of renal function, I have experience with the reviewing process, as I am asked at least three times per week to review a manuscript in my field. I reluctantly accept, because a thorough review takes about 3–4 hours' time which often is not available. You also do not receive any remuneration for your time. However,

© Springer Nature Switzerland AG 2019
G. Filler, R. Nagra, *Becoming a Successful Scholar*,
https://doi.org/10.1007/978-3-030-24448-4_12

it is still a great opportunity to help improve the quality of scientific publications, and the task also continually improves your own writing skills.

What exactly does reviewing entail? First and foremost, there is a big difference between reading and reviewing. When you read a scientific paper, you want to accrue that knowledge. Reading a scientific paper is for your own enrichment; for instance, if you are going to better understand the context and content of existing work in your field. Reviewing is very different. The goal is to assess the suitability of a scientific manuscript for the journal. Ideally, you should also assist in improving the manuscripts and enhancing its quality by giving a detailed assessment with suggestions for improvement.

Of course, as an editor, I have to review many manuscripts. Recently, some publishers have started to register the reviews. One of these, Publons, is a website and free service for academics to track, verify, and showcase their peer review and editorial contributions for academic journals. Publons was founded by Andrew Preston and Daniel Johnston to address the static state of peer-reviewing practices in academic research publishing. The hope is to encourage collaboration and speed up scientific development. The company is registered in New Zealand and was acquired last year by Clarivate Analytics, which is a company that produces excellent tools such as Web of Science, EndNote, and ScholarOne. Publons has partnerships with some major publishers, including Springer Nature, Oxford University Press, British Medical Journals, SAGE, Taylor and Francis, and Wiley. As I review a lot for transplant journals which are often housed by Wiley, about 50% of my reviews are captured on this website. As you can see in Fig. 12.1, my review activity may be a bit excessive.

Indeed, it is an excellent opportunity to learn and help authors, especially those from developing countries, to publish important findings which may otherwise be lost forever. As a reviewer, I read the manuscript ideally at least two times thoroughly and preferably a third time, although my time

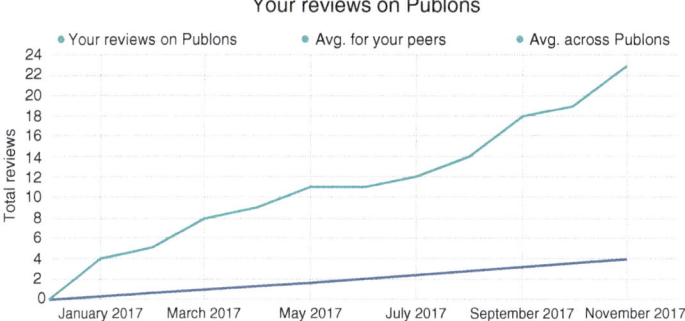

FIGURE 12.1 Reviews for scientific journals captured on Publons for 2017. Instead of an average of 4 reviews per researcher per year, I reviewed 23

constraints sometimes do not allow this. I have a word processor open to take notes as I read. The *methods*, *results*, as well as the *abstract* sections undoubtedly get a lot of attention. On the short paragraph about statistics, I sometimes spend 15 minutes. Sometimes I repeat some statistics to assess the plausibility. For a few years now, I have been keeping track of each review on the medical school's scientific activity website Acuity Star. As you can see in Fig. 12.2, about 30% of reviews take 4 hours. I had extensively edited manuscripts that I deemed important and sent the revised manuscript back together with the review, especially when I thought it was important to publish the findings. Unfortunately, you often do not get such thorough reviews. A reviewer may have a large number of papers to process and may not deeply be devoted to improving the content of any particular paper. Quite often, reviewers are chosen from the top leaders in a field, who have limited time and are already highly committed to their work. If you are lucky, you will get a diligent, thoughtful reviewer who provides thorough feedback, but do not be surprised if a review is not as comprehensive and meticulous as you would have liked or if the reviewer has

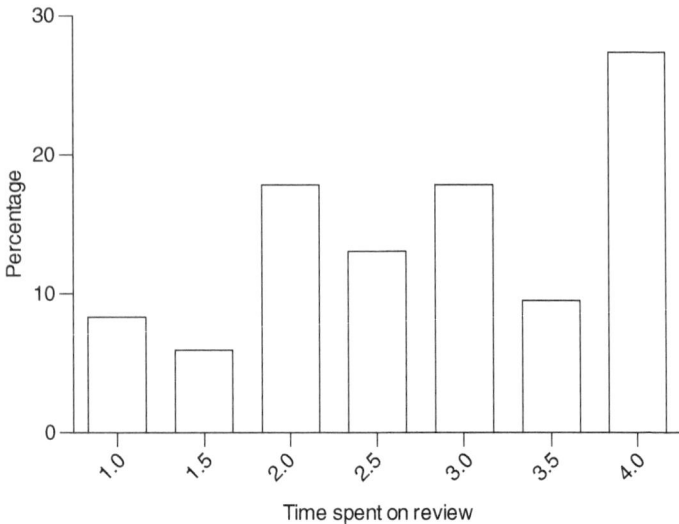

FIGURE 12.2 Length of time spent on reviews from 2015 to 2018

missed important points you were trying to make in your paper.

As an author, you should not be surprised if some of the comments seem trivial: there may be underlying issues of the current paradigm in a research field or personal preference that drove the reviewer's opinion on your paper that a reviewer may not explicitly state. Whenever I read reviews I receive for a rejected paper, I try to look past specifically detailed quibbles (or "excuses" for rejecting the paper) and figure out the big picture which may simply be that the reviewer could not find a reason to accept the paper. Especially when I have only one reviewer reject a paper and my own assessment is that the manuscript can be rescued, I may override the decision of the reviewer. Unfortunately, an editor often struggles to find a sufficient number of reviewers. She or he may not know any aspiring and upcoming experts in the field, and all too often we draw on the established leaders in the field. Fortunately, some of them pass the reviews on to some of their mentees. I strongly advise that you ask your supervisors to pass on their reviews to you and allow yourself to take on the role of a reviewer. During this process, you will have an opportunity to review your assessment with your supervisor, an incredible learning opportunity. Of course, this assumes that your supervisor reviews what you have written.

In your task of reviewing a paper, first and foremost, you should use a specific structure. I strongly recommend the checklists, such as CONSORT for randomized controlled clinical trials and STROBE for epidemiological studies. I always have a copy of the checklists open and mark the pages where I can find the appropriate information. Fortunately, some journals are now requiring a mandatory checklist to be submitted alongside the manuscript, which significantly helps to improve the manuscript. But more importantly than assessing adherence to form, which is just a tool for acquiring the necessary skill that you need to be able to assess the quality of a paper, you should ask some important questions and be able to find the answers from the paper. As suggested by Nick Feamster, they are (not necessarily in this order):

Does the Paper Realize a Great Idea?
- Is the problem important?
- Look for reason(s) to accept the paper. Does it realize a great contribution or idea?
- What makes the idea "great"?
- To what extent does the paper actually solve the problem it describes?
- Is there an intellectual contribution that is novel and/or outstanding?

Does the Main Conclusion Make Sense?
- What is the main contribution or conclusion and is it important?
- Does the content support the conclusions?
- Do the conclusions matter? "So what?"
- Are the findings generalizable?
- Are the limitations well described?

Is This Right for the Journal I Am Reviewing?
- Consider the audience, is the audience of the journal the most suitable audience for this paper?
- Consider the standards of the journal (this may well be the most tedious part of a review, but do check the reference style, the composition of the manuscript, structured abstract, etc.)
- Consider the purpose?

Consider the Big Picture!

This following paragraph by Dr. Feamster regarding the reviewing process is so spot on that I would like to cite it:

Every paper can be rejected. It is always easy to find reasons to reject a paper. The reviewer's goal should not be to identify the reasons to reject a paper, but rather to determine whether there are any reasons to accept the paper. If the answer to that question is negative, then it is always easy to find "excuses" to reject a paper. You should be aiming to figure out whether the paper has important contributions that the audience will benefit from knowing about, and whether the paper supports those contributions and conclusions to the level of standard that is commensurate with the standard of the audience and the venue. One *litmus test* I use to ensure that a negative aspect of a paper does not condemn it is to ask myself whether the problem (1) affects the main conclusion or contribution of the paper; and (2) can be fixed easily in a revision. If the problem doesn't alter the main contribution or conclusion, and if it can be easily fixed, then it should not negatively affect a paper's review [2].

Once you have answers to these questions, you are ready to write your review. Fortunately, most journals have a good template for the review, especially if they use the Manuscript Central websites. Start with a summary of the purpose and the merits of the paper. This should be a single and very concise paragraph. Then assess whether the paper delivers the main claims and contributions. Point out flaws, and include some judgment as to whether they are "fatal" like wrong starting hypotheses or the omission of significant confounders or whether they can be fixed. Focus on what the authors can do to fix the flaws in an itemized list. Occasionally, experiments may need to be completely redesigned because they fail to support any meaningful conclusion.

Even if you decide to reject the paper, please write something positive. These positive comments are not just for author morale (although that is important too): They give the author a direction to move forward. The worst reviews are those that reject a paper without providing any specific action for moving forward. The best reviews are those that highlight the positive aspects of the work while identifying weaknesses and areas where the work could be further developed to overcome weaknesses or problems. Write about the paper, not the authors. Consider what kind of feedback you would like to receive when writing your review. Always be polite and focus on suggestions for improvement. I do recommend that you seek an opportunity to review a manuscript at least once per month, incorporate the advice named above, and you will soon learn how to write a manuscript from the eyes of a reviewer. Perhaps the most critical skill to have for becoming a successful author is to know what comprises a good manuscript and how to write it. Believe me, working as a reviewer is your best avenue to achieve these skills. Do not consider reviewing as "working for free" but rather as an opportunity to sharpen your own skills. Remember what Covey said about sharpening the saw? Reviewing is "sharpening the saw"! Do not be a fool and miss this chance by thinking you are too busy to review a manuscript. Actively seek out opportunities to review, be it through your supervisor or through contacting experts in your field and offering them to assist them with their review activities.

References

1. https://greatresearch.org/2013/10/18/the-paper-reviewing-process/.
2. https://greatresearch.org/2013/10/18/the-paper-reviewing-process/.

Chapter 13
The Road to Success

My favorite book is called *Momo*, by Michael Ende. This is the same author who wrote *The Neverending Story*. It is a children's book. *Momo*, also known as *The Grey Gentlemen*, is a fantasy novel by Michael Ende, published in 1973, and later was made into a movie. It is about the concept of time and how humans use it in modern societies. The full title in German (Momo oder Die seltsame Geschichte von den Zeit-Dieben und von dem Kind, das den Menschen die gestohlene Zeit zurückbrachte) translates to "the strange story of the time thieves and the child who brought the stolen time back to the people." What fascinated me even as a child was not the hero, Momo, who is this mystery girl that lives in an amphitheater in an unnamed city (although it seems like Southern Italy, perhaps Positano or Amalfi) but rather her friend Beppo.

Momo does not know how old she is or how she came to the ruins. She is illiterate and cannot count, parentless and wearing a long, used coat. She is remarkable in the neighborhood because she has the extraordinary ability to listen – really listen. By simply being with people and listening to them, she can help them find answers to their problems, make up with each other, and think of fun games. The advice which was given to people "go and see Momo!" becomes a common phrase, and Momo makes many friends, especially her honest, silent street cleaner, Beppo.

© Springer Nature Switzerland AG 2019
G. Filler, R. Nagra, *Becoming a Successful Scholar*,
https://doi.org/10.1007/978-3-030-24448-4_13

The arrival of the Men in Grey eventually revealed as a species of paranormal parasites stealing the time of humans destroys the pleasant atmosphere. Appearing in the form of grey-clad, grey-skinned, bald men, these strange individuals present themselves as representing the Timesavings Bank and promote the idea of "timesaving" among the population: supposedly, time can be deposited in the Bank and returned to the client later with interest. After encountering the Men in Grey, people are made to forget all about them, but not about the resolution to save as much time as possible with the result life becomes sterile, devoid of all things considered time-wasting, like social activities, recreation, art, imagination, or sleeping. Buildings and clothing are made precisely the same for everyone, and the rhythms of life become hectic. Momo eventually rescues the town from these grey men. However, I do not want to give away the plot and will instead focus on Beppo.

Beppo is old and has gout, arthritis, and a job sweeping the streets. When he gets his assignments and sees the long winding road all the way down to the valley and up again to the next hill, he might as well have given up on this overwhelming feat. But he does not do that. He looks at the first tile and cuts it into an imaginary half. He then sweeps the first half and then the second half, now on to the next tile, also divided into two halves, and so on. Before the day is done, he has swept the long winding road all the way down the valley and up the hill, and he does not even remember how he did it.

The lesson from this approach is that every journey starts with one step. Think only of the first step and do that step well, then on to the next step, and so on. Before you know it, you have completed your entire assignment, no matter how insurmountable it had seemed before. If you get impressed with its towering imposing demeanor, you might as well give up. Do not do that. Cut the first tile into an imaginary half. Focus on that half alone, and work your way to the next one. Every journey starts with one step. Got it?

Chapter 14
Your Future Road to Success

Research can be fun! It is a privilege to work in an academic health sciences center or institution that pays you to do research. Your mindset will determine everything. Do not consider the privilege of communicating your teachable moments as a burden but rather as an opportunity.

I hope I have shown you what you need to think only about the next step and work at a steady pace at your particular 17-mile march intervals. What your 17-mile march is you have to determine for yourself. But do it every day. Jim Collins calls that fanatic discipline.

Do not fire your cannonballs at once. Consider small pilot projects with resource consumption that is expendable before writing your big grant proposal or making the huge research investment. If the bullets did not hit their mark, what is the point of firing the final cannonball? Jim Collins calls that empirical creativity.

Also, schedule and plan. As outlined, you do not do your residency learning in the last 3 months before your exam. Your mind just does not work like that. It needs steady, regular input to gradually accrue new knowledge and new skills. Pace your work. Work with a buffer. Work well above the death line. Jim Collins calls this productive paranoia.

Finally, do not dwell on potential luck. It is not the luck that makes us successful but the return on luck.

© Springer Nature Switzerland AG 2019   133
G. Filler, R. Nagra, *Becoming a Successful Scholar*,
https://doi.org/10.1007/978-3-030-24448-4_14

Everything that Jim Collins proposes that makes companies in times of high change resilient can be applied to you as a person.

Use the power of habits to automate your work, instead of relying on motivation. For instance, do the most challenging task of the day first thing in the morning to boost your productivity. Do not procrastinate. Divide your work appropriately, so your mind perceives more than a 70% likelihood for success of the task. Use the principles of influence such as reciprocity, and commitment and consistency, rather than authority to drive your work. Work in a team. Use your outlined expectations from your peers for your assignments to help keep you on track.

I hope I have shown you that research can be fun and that you have to give it a lot of structure. You need to *zoom out* to design the big template, then go into details, and make your MeisterTask list (or whatever program you choose to use). Work in Steven Covey's Quadrant 2: important but not urgent. Do not indulge in trivia or social media; they are just not important! See the long-term goal, but think only of the next step.

Consider the growth psychology. We are here to live to the best of our potential. You already have Level 5 ambition, and you should be proud of it. But pace yourself and consider the advice above. This should lead you to success. Now, we wish you happy researching!

Index

© Springer Nature Switzerland AG 2019
G. Filler, R. Nagra, *Becoming a Successful Scholar*,
https://doi.org/10.1007/978-3-030-24448-4